From
Julia Nelle Grandle

POT OF GOLD

POT
OF
GOLD

Julia Nelle Grandle

VANTAGE PRESS
New York / Washington / Atlanta
Los Angeles / Chicago

FIRST EDITION

Published by Vantage Press, Inc.
516 West 34th Street, New York, New York 10001

Manufactured in the United States of America
ISBN: 0-533-06370-1

Library of Congress Catalog Card No.: 84-90490

To my husband Jimmy and our wonderful family

Foreword

For many years, I have felt that I wanted to write the story of our experiences in living with a child who has a visible handicap. It has been my hope in writing this story that those who read it will come to realize, as I have, that each child is born a unique being. One is born with a handicap that can be easily detected. . . . another is born with a handicap not visible to the casual observer . . . but within his makeup, something will be a handicap that must be overcome.

Love, care, and understanding help the child to develop the strength and the determination to overcome whatever handicap he may have, and to grow into a useful, happy adult who will take his place in his community with pride and satisfaction. It is God who creates, and He, who has a plan for each child. His guiding hand is forever with him, even though, at times, He seems to work in very mysterious ways. At times it is very hard for a parent to accept this. . . . For sometimes His plan calls for His "little angels" to come to live with Him before they have a chance to know much about the life on this earth.

Whatever His plan . . . our family has been given the opportunity to share the joys of living with three of His children . . . one with a visible handicap. This is the story that follows.

Acknowledgments

I am very grateful for the help of my friends Nancy Stewart and Dianne Fertitta in preparing my manuscript for publication.

POT
OF
GOLD

I

I could hardly see to focus my camera. I kept trying to push back the tears that seemed to be welling up in my eyes. These were tears of joy and pride. There I stood, in the mass of humanity, viewing a scene that I had witnessed at least five times before. This year the weather was ideal. It was a lovely spring day to stand under the broad spreading maples and oaks which lined the lawn planned by Thomas Jefferson so many years before.

We had arrived very early for the graduation ceremony. Experience had taught us that if we were to find a spot where we could place chairs for the grandmothers to see the academic procession, we would have to get there several hours ahead of the time that the procession was to begin. Our older sons had joined me in wandering through the crowd to be sure that we had the best view for our cameras. I had found a spot just a few feet from the roped-off area near one of the many sets of steps leading down the terraced lawn. I had managed to make arrangements with those who were standing closer, to let me get in front of them when my son came down those particular steps.

The band had been playing for some time; finally, the trumpeters marched up the Lawn to lead the procession down the long walk to the front of Cabbell Hall, where the graduation exercises would take place.

Excitedly, I watched what seemed to be thousands of black-robed figures in cap and gown, four abreast, come down the steps. Each school was designated by a different color of tassel. Bright orange was the color of the Engineering School, but other schools also had shades of orange. Several times I asked to stand out in front so that I might take the picture that I so very much wanted. Each time it was the wrong group.

Finally, I spotted the Dean of the School of Engineering and Applied Sciences; I knew then that I would get my picture soon. The threat of the tears in my eyes suddenly caused twenty-three years to pass quickly across my mind.

Oddly, just thirty hours short of exactly twenty-three years before this graduation, Jimmy, my wonderful husband, and two doctors had stood in my hospital room with tears in their eyes as they told me about our newly born son. What they had been saying did not have much meaning for me. I had never heard the words "spina bifida" before that time. I felt that I couldn't cry; I had to be brave, to give Jimmy strength. Actually, I guess that I was still too much under the influence of the sedative to realize just what had been said to me.

Earlier that Sunday, Jimmy, the boys, and I had attended church, and after the usual Sunday afternoon nap, settled on the front porch for our favorite pastime of car watching. This Sunday was different, because my mother was not with us as had been her custom since my father's passing almost a year before. She had decided to go with my aunt and uncle to visit a friend in Maryland.

As I sat there enjoying my family and the lovely spring day, I had a feeling of satisfaction and happiness. I had been able to find a lovely young girl named Gerry Deavers to help me get my annual spring cleaning completed, and she had agreed to return to stay with us while I was hospitalized for the birth of our third child, an event I felt would not be too far in the future.

Suddenly a sharp pain hit me. I was a bit suspicious. In about five minutes I had another pain, and then I knew that it was about time to call the doctor. He said that I should "come on" to the hospital and he would meet me there. Jimmy was worried about leaving the boys, but they said that they would be good. Jimmy said that he would try to call Gerry from the hospital to come to stay with them until he got home. I assured him that I didn't think that I would have a long labor since this was our third child.

The doctor arrived at the hospital shortly after I was admitted. He said that he felt that I would not deliver for at least several hours, so he would go have his dinner, then return. I learned later that his dinner had been interrupted. I delivered a son within the hour.

The next morning, the sedative that I had been given was gone. I was full of questions. Surely there must be some mistake. The nurses who came and went were very cautious. They were overly cheerful in their greetings. After what seemed to be hours, my obstetrician and the pediatrician who cared for our children appeared together at my door.

Both seemed very serious and, almost before I could ask if our son was still living, they almost jointly blurted out that he had made it through the night. Questions were flying through my head in such rapid fashion that I didn't know which ones to ask first. I heard myself blurting out: "What is the term that you used last night for the baby's condition?" I couldn't seem to remember anything from the night before except the tears in Jimmy's eyes and the look of concern on the faces of these two men now sitting by my bed.

Dr. George repeated the words "spina bifida." Then he drew a prescription pad from his pocket and started to draw a picture of the spinal column. He was explaining to me how the vertebrae are, more or less, round with a hollow center through which the spinal cord passes. It seems that in some babies, in our baby, the vertebrae are open—they do not form a complete circle and the spinal cord and the nerves that grow out from it develop through the hole. The spinal cord fails to develop through the vertebrae below that point, thus causing the lower parts of the body to develop without nerves, the body's vital communication links to the brain.

Dr. Calhoun explained that many of the children who are born with this condition do not live more than a few days.

There are many dangers. Some develop infections, hydrocephalus, or urinary infections.

My next question was "When can I see him?" Both men avoided a direct answer, but they tried to satisfy me with a promise that they would see how my condition and the baby's condition developed in the next few days. They both warned that I should not become too hopeful. They just did not see how Baby Grandle could survive.

Dr. George said that he wanted me to sit up and to walk around in my room, but not to do more than go to the bathroom for that day. He would give me medication to dry up my milk that might develop in my breasts. I almost laughed, for I had tried to nurse our first two children; in spite of the fact that I am well-endowed, I just did not produce enough milk to feed the guys. I told him that I didn't think I would have to worry about milk, judging from my previous pregnancies. Wouldn't you know: this time I did have milk for the baby, and for several days it caused me some discomfort.

Visiting hours were very limited, but I somehow managed to fight off the terrible loneliness and depression that kept swelling up inside of me. I did call my mother to check on how she was and see if the boys were all right with Gerry. She assured me that all were fine. She planned to come by during the visiting hours in the afternoon.

Jimmy wouldn't be able to come by until after supper that evening, for he had responsibilities that he needed to attend to at work. He was employed as the assistant manager of a turkey hatchery that was owned by a friend of ours. As much as I felt that I wanted him near, I knew that it was best for him to go about his daily work so that he did not have time to worry.

I was really surprised when Jimmy managed to slip in shortly before lunch, even though no visitors were allowed until midafternoon. I think that the nurses turned their heads so that they wouldn't see him slip into my room. He was much calmer by that time. Mostly we sat and held each other's hand. Somehow, we knew that we must give this child of ours a name, because he was a living soul and our flesh and blood. We could not have him die without a name.

During the months that I had carried this life within me, I had said we should name this child either Christopher or Christina. The older son, named after his father, was called Art, a shortened form of Arthur—his middle name—to avoid the confusion of having two Jimmys in the family. The next son was named Robert and we called him Bob. The boys, only thirteen months apart in age, had, for many years, been almost the same size. I used to mark their clothes with their initials, A and B. People would tease Jimmy and ask if he were working on the alphabet. It seemed that our third child should be given a name that began with *C*.

Jimmy agreed that Christopher seemed like a good name, and I suggested the given name of my mother's brother, Owen. So the decision was made. The third son of James Arthur Grandle and Julia Nelle Blosser Grandle would be named Christopher Owen Grandle. We would call him Chris. This was also the name of Jimmy's grandfather Grandle.

I made a weak attempt at reporting to Jimmy the things that Dr. George and Dr. Calhoun had told me earlier. It was so hard. There were so many things that neither of us understood. I wanted him to stay there with me, but I knew that he had work to do and had to get back to the hatchery.

The boys told me later that they had been so worried about their dad the night that Chris was born. They reported that it was the first time that they had ever seen him cry.

My room was beginning to be filled with beautiful flowers sent by our friends. I think that the single yellow rose from my sorority sisters meant the most to me. The flowers lined the wide windowsill—over them I had a lovely view of the magnificent Shenandoah Valley with the Blue Ridge Mountains in the background. Looking out over the beauty that God created, I could not help but wonder why He had made our Chris something less than perfect.

I kept repeating a silent prayer that Chris might live: "God, help me to understand or at least to accept your plan for this child that I have borne."

Dr. Calhoun dropped by, just before the afternoon visiting hours, to say that Chris was still living, but that he had developed a fever and it looked as if he was getting weaker. He was taking some milk at each feeding. The doctor went on to tell me that there was so little known about these children. I got the feeling from what he was telling me that he really hoped Chris would not live too long. I got the idea that in the rare event that when these children had survived, they were primarily vegetation. They could not sit up, their heads grew large, and their backs curved so that the head pulled backward, almost touching the feet.

I understood what was being said to me and I repeated it later that evening to Jimmy and my mother, but I could not believe or accept what the words were expressing. Even the worst things that I had studied and read in the college psychology class years before had not seemed that grotesque. Yet, I knew Dr. Calhoun so well and had a great deal of faith in him. He had treated our older boys since birth. He had taken over the practice of my own beloved childhood doctor. How could I not believe what he was telling me?

After evening visiting hours ended, the nurse brought my pills and gave me a comforting backrub. Then I was all alone in the dark. I felt hot tears welling in my eyes, and again I prayed for acceptance of God's plan, whatever it might be. One of the pills must have been a sleeping pill of some sort, for it was not long before I found myself drifting off to sleep.

The next morning, Dr. Calhoun arrived early. Chris had had several convulsions during the night and his fever was higher than it had been the day before. He felt that the fever was causing the convulsions, but he could only guess at the cause of the fever. Things did not look good.

Dr. George stopped by for just a few minutes, but he did say that he anticipated letting me go home on Thursday, unless something unforeseen should come up.

The rest of that day and the next were much the same:

Jimmy and Mom came in as much as they could, friends called, nurses stopped by for friendly small talk. On Wednesday evening, my brother, Henry, and his wife came from Charlottesville and asked at the nursery to see Chris. Apparently, someone neglected to tell a student nurse on duty not to show Baby Grandle. Henry met Mother and Jimmy outside the hospital; he related that they had seen Chris and that he was a beautiful baby. When Mom told me, my first question was, had he seen the baby's feet and legs? Mom didn't think to ask, and the family was on their way back to Charlottesville.

Thursday morning, Dr. Calhoun made his usual stop by the room. He still had nothing good to report, except the convulsions seemed to have stopped and the fever was not quite as high. He thought that it might be a good idea to X-ray Chris. I told him that I would be going home that day, and I almost pleaded with him to let me at least see Chris before I left the hospital. I really didn't think it fair that Henry had seen my baby and I couldn't. Dr. Calhoun tried to explain, he didn't want me to become more attached to the baby, because he felt that losing him would just be harder on me. Finally, I did get him to say that I could call the nursery each day to find out how he was getting along.

Jimmy was there to take me home about eleven, just as he had promised. Dr. George warned me to take it easy, not to drive, or go up and down steps for at least three weeks. I had been prepared for this advice; Gerry and I had fixed my temporary bed in the den while we were in the process of spring cleaning.

It was good to be home, to be with the boys and their lively activities, to be able to help plan meals and begin to be involved in the routine of running our home. Gerry proved to be a good companion, and our relation blossomed into a lasting friendship. She helped me a great deal in those first days at home. She seemed to be able to sense when I wanted to talk, or when I would just rather sit on the porch, watching the cars and people go by. I'm sure that the personnel in the nursery at the hospital became very tired of my calling and asking how Chris was doing. Three times a day, I called. Sometimes his fever went down, and they thought that maybe, just maybe, he was a little stronger; then his fever went up again and he was not so well. Those wonderful nurses never let me know they were troubled by my calling. Each time I called, they patiently reported Chris's condition.

Now that I was home, and Jimmy could embrace me in his arms, I could no longer restrain the tears. That first night at home, we both wept until there were no more tears. We had looked forward to having this child to spoil and to love. Not that we didn't love the older boys, for we did, very much; yet Art, born in the first year of our marriage, was quite young when I found that I was pregnant again. Jimmy and I had married very young. He was about to go overseas when we were married. I, a sophomore in college, had promised my parents that I would finish my schooling. I finished four years of college in three years. Our second son, Bob, was born just two months after I finished school. During the first six years of our married life, we lived with my parents. They wanted to help us get started after Jimmy was discharged from service at the end of the war. We have always appreciated their help during that time, and during the building of our home. Still, living with parents was not the same as living in a place of our own.

Now, after nine years, we were in our own home; Bob was almost eight years old. We had really wanted this third child. The boys, too, had been very excited about having a new baby in the house. A baby brother's birth was something that neither of them had really ever experienced. Art was so young when Bob arrived on the scene that he could not remember what it was like not to have a brother. We had all worked in getting the old baby furniture out of Mother's attic and refinishing it. The bassinet, one that I had slept in, had been used when the boys were born. Bob had picked at the woven sides until he had a large hole in the panels. We had to have this rewoven before we put on the white paint and the lovely decals that the boys had helped me to select at the five-and-ten.

Before I had come home from the hospital, Jimmy and Gerry had very carefully put the bed back in Mother's attic. They had put away all of the diapers and lovely baby clothes that I had collected. I didn't bother to ask what had happened to them. . . . I really didn't care.

Even though I became involved in running the house and in reading, I realized the days were long during that first week. I decided that it wouldn't hurt me to go to church the first Sunday I was home. There were just two steps at our back door and only three at the front door of the church. I very much wanted to go. Jimmy agreed that the trip probably would not hurt me if I took it slow and easy. He was able to find a place to park right at the front door of the church. We sat on the back bench. Very few people knew that we were there, because we slipped out before the service concluded. I felt as though I didn't want to talk to a lot of people.

Day followed day during that second week. Things were pretty much the same. One day Chris would be better, and the next day worse. When good days seemed to outnumber the bad ones, I became a little brighter. The heaviness that I had felt continually in my heart was lifting somewhat.

My brother, Henry, was to receive his Ph.D. from the University of Virginia that next weekend. I very much wanted to attend the graduation exercise. I called Dr. George. I told him that I felt fine. I insisted that I would not walk a great deal and that I would avoid all steps. Finally, he agreed to my going to Charlottesville. It was good for me to get away, to have a change, and to see people that did not know me and our Chris. We could talk about what was happening at the moment.

The days of the third week seemed to run together. All of the calls to the nursery gave me much the same information each day. There was a growing desire in me to see and to hold Chris in my arms. Each day that he lived added a new spark of hope that maybe . . . just maybe . . . Dr. Calhoun and Dr. George could be wrong.

On Monday of the fourth week, I felt a surge of panic rush over me when I made my regular call to the nusery. At the other end of the line a voice that I had not heard before was telling me that Baby Grandle was no longer in the nursery. What had happened? Was he still living? Where had they taken him? The questions came out in a great rush.

Chris had been moved to the pediatrics floor. The nursery did not have room for him any longer, and he was getting too big for the facilities there. Dr. Calhoun called shortly to tell me that the move had been made. I could continue calling for information. I was familiar with the hospital regulations, so, knowing that there were regular afternoon visiting hours, I did not ask about the possibility of visiting Chris. I persuaded my mother to take me that afternoon to the hospital to see Chris for the first time. I was almost afraid; yet, I knew that I just had to see him.

In pediatrics, Gloria, a student nurse assigned to care for Chris, was so loving and wonderful to both of us. It was just as Henry had said! Chris was a beautiful baby. When Gloria handed him to me, he looked just like any other three-week-old baby, wrapped gently in a very light blue receiving blanket. Gloria cautioned me to be very careful of his back as I held him. Dr. Calhoun had shown me, in his drawings, that there was a sack of some sort on Chris's back where the nerves had grown out of his spinal cord. With fear, and trembling, I asked Gloria if I could take off the blanket to look at the rest of his body.

Gently, Gloria helped me unfold the blanket. There, I saw for the first time, those little froglike legs with the little misshapen feet. His toes were bent around so that they almost touched his heels. They were rosy and soft like the feet of any baby. In spite of what I saw, I felt relieved, for I had imagined all kinds of terrible things. I held the little feet in my hand. They were still and motionless. How could anyone help but love this beautiful child? Gently, I wrapped the blanket back as I talked to this bright child who seemed to know exactly what I was saying. Gloria remarked at how well he could hold up his hand. I avoided asking to see his back during this first trip. Visiting hours were limited to fifteen minutes per patient. I decided to come back the next day and each day that someone would drive me during that week.

On my second visit to the pediatrics floor I got up enough courage to ask Gloria to show me Chris's back. It was covered with sterile dressings secured with a "belly band." The danger of infection in this area was probably the greatest danger that faced this small child of ours. There, on his back, I saw a large lump about the size of a turkey egg, covered with folds of reddish skin that looked very much like the skin of a mole. A clear fluid slowly oozed from between the folds of skin. This was the spinal fluid that was getting to the surface. A clean sterile bandage was quickly applied and secured after Gloria gently bathed the meningocele with a saline solution.

Each day, as I visited Chris, I looked for signs that hydrocephalus might be developing, but I could not see any indications. True, Chris had a head that seemed to be larger than some of the other children in the ward, but both of his brothers, Art and Bob, had had large heads when they were born. I did not see anything unusual in the size of Chris's head. He was so bright and alert. I just did not see how there was even a possibility of any hydrocephalus.

During the fourth week after Chris's birth, Dr. Calhoun called me. He was concerned that I had been visiting Chris on such a regular basis. Again, he mentioned the heartbreak that he felt was sure to come when we lost Chris. By this time, I had accepted the fact that God must have some plan. Although I was not to know or to understand, I perceived that He would help us through whatever came. I wanted to be with Chris and to love him as much as time would allow.

About this same time I received a wonderful gift from my namesake who lived in Arizona. It was a small book by Dale Evans—*Angel Unaware.* I must have read that little book several times. It helped me to realize that we were not the first to have a child who is less than perfect. It made me see that God has a plan for each of us. Maybe Chris would be another of His "little angels" or maybe God had planned some other work for him. Those possibilities did not have to be answered for me. . . . I knew that He would always be with us and guide us.

One day, shortly after my talk with Dr. Calhoun, Gloria agreed to help me set up the lights of our movie camera and take some pictures of Chris. Even then he was a true camera "hog." He laughed and smiled, cooed and "talked" to Gloria, as I took the pictures. Dr. Calhoun found out about this later and honestly thought that I shouldn't have done it. I'm so glad that we did! They turned out well, considering the fact that we had poor light and I didn't know much about the camera.

During the fifth week, Dr. Calhoun suggested that we consider moving Chris to a small nursing home that he knew about in New Market. He said that the lady in charge was very kind and made a specialty of caring for "afflicted" children. Chris did not seem to be running a fever anymore and Dr. Calhoun felt that our son could probably live as long as ten months. Already the hospital expenses were great, and the facilities were inadequate to continue to care for him. In the doctor's opinion, the hydrocephalus would probably begin to develop more rapidly as he became a few months older, and this was a condition our older boys should not see. They were at an age when this development would be hard to explain or accept. We agreed.

On Thursday, it was decided that we would take Dr. Calhoun's suggestion. We felt that we would like to have Chris baptized before we took him to the nursing home. I called our pastor, Rev. Swain, to see if arrangements could be made for a private baptism on Sunday afternoon. He was most cooperative and willing to do anything that we wanted.

I spent Friday looking through the store, hunting for a white suit that Chris could wear, something that would not be too tight over his back. I found and purchased a beautiful little white nylon suit. I planned to wrap a lovely blue-and-white shawl around him.

So, on Sunday afternoon, the Fourth of July, Jimmy and I went by the hospital to get Chris. We left Bob and Art waiting excitedly in the car. As I slipped into the front seat with Chris in my arms, the boys were pushing and shoving to get the most advantageous position to see him.

Rev. Swain was waiting for us at the church. He led the five of us into the quiet sanctuary, where we stood before the altar as he read the baptismal service. Christopher Owen Grandle received the rite of baptism on the day which marked the sixth week since his birth.

Several of the shrubs around the outside of the church were in bloom, and we thought that they would make a nice background for a family portrait. Rev. Swain helped in taking the picture so we could all be included. I had to push the boys away from trying to touch Chris. They wanted to get close to him and to place their hands on him. Finally, after the picture taking, each of them was allowed to sit, holding Chris for a few minutes. Then we dropped them off at home with Gerry, while Jimmy and I made the long, long, eighteen-mile drive to New Market.

We took the back roads and drove very slowly. Chris seemed to be enjoying the ride, and we enjoyed having him with us. Just before we got to the town limits of New Market. I decided that we should stop to take some pictures. We found a large shade tree by the side of the road, and here we pulled off for the picture taking. However, Chris had found that riding made him sleepy, so he really was not interested in the camera. I tried to get him awake without much success.

There was a very small sign outside of the large, old, brick home on the main street of New Market. The house did not seem to be in the best state of repair, but I noticed that it was spotless. A large, jolly woman met us at the door and introduced herself as Mrs. Henkel, the proprietress. She led us into the room on the left, where several other infants lay in cribs. They seemed to be happy and well tended. Mrs. Henkel talked to them as she took Chris from me, telling the other infants that they had a new roommate, and making the introductions as though they knew exactly what she was saying. It was obvious that she loved children.

I felt satisfied that Chris would receive good care and lots of love. I left him without a feeling of apprehension. During the weeks to come, I was to learn more about Mrs. Henkel and the nursing home which she operated.

II

It was about this time that Gerry left us to go help another new mother. I, once again, took over the full-time management of my home and family. Time was not as abundant as it had been. I managed somehow to make the time to go to New Market on Monday, Wednesday, and Friday. Then, on Sunday afternoon, all of the family went. I tried to arrange my visits so that Chris would not be taking a nap or eating. I didn't always miss the naps. Sometimes, I would just sit and watch him while he slept, and I would talk to Mrs. Henkel. She told about how she was massaging his feet, trying to get them to straighten up. She had even put a small pair of shoes on his feet. She had put them on the wrong feet because she felt that might help. I didn't know how effective the practice might be, but certainly it didn't seem to hurt anything. . . . She might help him.

During those times when we talked, I learned that Mrs. Henkel was a midwife. She took care of many of the mountain women who refused or could not afford to go to the hospital for the birth of their children. They came to her nursing home. She also took care of many unwed mothers, often taking care of the baby until adoption could be arranged by the welfare department. The right side of the hallway, which we had entered that first day, led to the maternity "ward" of three hospital beds. She had a delivery room set up in an adjoining room. I was always amazed at how clean she managed to keep everything. Mrs. Henkel was the only cook and bottle-washer,

her sole help being her eleven-year-old adopted daughter. She fed and clothed the four babies who were her patients. She delivered babies and cared for the mothers until they were strong enough to return home. On most of the sunny days, she found the time, in the late evening, to take Chris out for a stroll in the old baby carriage which she kept on the back porch.

I was amazed that anyone could do so much. The even more amazing thing was that she furnished all of the food, clothing, and care, for only one dollar per day. True, she did not have the nice equipment of a hospital, but her equipment, though old, was adequate for what she did. No equipment or money could have given the love that she provided for each of her patients.

The opening on Chris's back was exposed when we took him to New Market. It was still necessary to cover it with the sterile dressing and to clean it with the saline solution. Mrs. Henkel noticed that the drainage was becoming less each day. Both of us were watching for signs for the dreaded hydrocephalus. Frequently, we checked the size of his head with a tape measure, but no rapid or unusual change occurred.

There was a small porch on the front of the New Market house. On each side, next to a railing, was a neatly painted white bench. The boys and I enjoyed many lazy summer afternoons sitting on those benches, taking turns holding Chris. Sometimes, we rocked him in the big, old-fashioned, high-backed rocker on the porch. It took up almost all of the porch space. We had to stop rocking if someone wanted to get in or out of the front door.

On Sunday afternoons, we took Chris in the car and rode through the shady back streets of the little, old-fashioned town. I always held Chris, the boys in the back seat hanging over so that they could see every move Chris made with his little hands or every expression that he had on his face. They wanted to be sure that they didn't miss anything. Chris seemed to be noticing their moves and reacted to them, delighting the boys.

We always carried a folding chair or two in the car, so

we sometimes stopped under a shady tree, got out, just sat, and enjoyed being together as a family. The camera was usually with us and in use. Mostly we took movies. For these Sunday afternoon occasions, Mrs. Henkel dressed Chris in one of the little diaper shirts I had gotten for him as a part of his layette.

After about three weeks at Mrs. Henkel's, Chris apparently had no spinal fluid draining from his back. I reported this cessation to Dr. Calhoun, who was concerned that this stoppage would cause the pressure to build up and to cause the enlarging of the head. He told me to keep an accurate record of the measurements that we were making of his head. I continued to insist that Chris's head was no larger than Bob's had been when he was the same age, but no proof existed except a mother's knowledge of her child. Doctors do not find that to be very scientific evidence.

Mrs. Henkel was confident that the massaging of the feet and legs was helping. The measurements were taken and records were kept. By the end of the fifth week, Dr. Calhoun was beginning to accept my point of view. He felt that maybe something could be done. He decided to call a doctor who he knew at Johns Hopkins University Hospital in Baltimore. Soon, he called back to tell me the doctor was out of the country for the summer, but that he had made arrangements for another doctor to see Chris. We had an appointment in Baltimore on August 23. We had to have Chris there by 1:00 P.M.

July and August are the busiest times of the year for a turkey hatchery. At that time, the poults are hatched that will be ready for the Thanksgiving and Christmas market. Jimmy said that he did not see how he could get away to go to Baltimore, so Mother volunteered to take Chris and me. The boys planned to ride along with her, and they would return the same afternoon. Dr. Calhoun said that the hospital would probably keep Chris at least a week to run a battery of tests.

We figured that the drive would take about four and a half hours or maybe even five. We told Mrs. Henkel that we expected to pick Chris up a little after seven. I had borrowed a car bed from a friend, so that Chris could ride more comfortably. I also felt that the car bed would free me to do some, or most of, the driving. I was concerned that the round trip might be too much for Mom. However, she often drove great distances by herself.

Chris was ready and waiting for us when we pulled up at the front door of the old house. Mrs. Henkel had fixed several bottles of formula for Chris. I also had borrowed a diaper bag with a few new diapers, so we began the journey confidently.

As we rode along to Baltimore, it dawned on me that Chris was celebrating his birthday. He was three months old that day, and he seemed to like traveling. We stopped once to give him a bottle and make a necessary change. A full stomach put him to sleep for a while.

With a map and one stop for directions, we found Johns Hopkins without much difficulty. After Mom and the boys had seen Chris admitted to the hospital, we said good-bye, and they started out for the return trip home.

I remember not being at all impressed by the appearance of this world-renowned medical center. The building was old—something that reminded me of the Victorian era—high ceilings, plastered archways, wooden floors, and wide stairways. All of the walls were painted a sort of sickening shade of green. I remember some places where the cracked plaster had not been repaired.

After admittance, I followed a nurse down the hall to a room containing two cribs. She indicated that I should put Chris in the one next to the window. There was one straight chair at the foot of the bed. There I sat for hours, waiting . . . waiting for a doctor to come to see Chris and to get the tests under way. A nurse came in, occasionally, to bring a bottle or a stack of diapers. Each time I asked if she had any idea when the doctor would be in. She didn't seem to know anything . . . even why we were there.

About midafternoon, a new set of nurses appeared. I inquired about a place where I might rent a room for the next several nights. One of the nurses told me that she had a room in a home near the hospital, and she would call to see if she could make arrangements for me to stay there. She was successful, and said that when I was ready to leave the hospital she would give me directions. I was told I would have to leave at 5:00 P.M. I could return the next morning at 10:00 A.M.

The nurses assured me that they would take good care of Chris. They showed me the way to the small snack bar across the court in the hospital, where I could get something to eat. In spite of the fact I usually require nourishment at regular times to keep going, I did not feel very hungry. I felt alone and scared.

I found my way to the room that I was to occupy for the night or the next week. It was small and hot. The window opened onto the street. It was hard to get to sleep. I lay there thinking and wondering if maybe the doctor had seen Chris after I left the hospital. Or what if he visited him in the morning before I was allowed in? Again, I felt the tears come into my eyes. Please, dear God, show this doctor what to do for Chris.

I was up early and had breakfast long before ten o'clock. I spent the time wandering around the brick-paved sidewalks near the hospital. I walked down near a construction site and watched the men working. I must have stood there amost an hour.

When the magic hour of 10:00 A.M. arrived, I was waiting outside the door leading into the pediatrics ward where the nurses had put Chris the day before. I was anxious to talk to the nurse to see if the doctor had been in. All of the nurses seemed to be flying here, there, and everywhere, with not a minute to stop and to answer my burning questions. Finally, as I sat on that hard, straight chair at the side of Chris's bed, a nurse came in and I found out that the doctor had not yet seen Chris. Was anything going to be done for him? No! Not until the doctor had a chance to examine him.

I sat a while; I paced the floor. I checked my watch. Yes, it was running. The time would soon be noon, and still no doctor. What was keeping him? Why had they told us to be there almost twenty-four hours ago? They hadn't even so much as looked at Chris! Couldn't the nurse call and find out about when I could expect the doctor? Yes, the doctor was in the hospital and he would be by as soon as he could get here.

One o'clock . . . still no doctor . . . my stomach was beginning to tell me that I needed some kind of nourishment. I began to feel weak and a little weary. I could slip across the courtyard, get a coke, and be back in less than ten minutes. I looked out in the hall to see anybody who looked as if he might be Chris's doctor. There were only young interns standing around talking to some of the nurses at the nurses' station. I surely could get to the snack bar and back. I hurried down those wide wooden steps, across the hall, out the door, across the courtyard, and into the shop. The snack shop was almost deserted and I had my coke in a few minutes. I sat at the counter, drinking it hurriedly. I began retracing my steps to the second floor where Chris's room was located.

As I started up the steps, I saw a middle-aged man of medium build, with a round face, start down the steps toward me. I knew the instant that I saw him that he was a doctor. Fear went through me. . . . Was he the doctor that was to see Chris? Had he been there, and had I missed him?

Suddenly, we were face-to-face on the steps, and I heard myself saying, "Are you Dr. Cantrell? I'm Mrs. Grandle."

"Yes, I'm Dr. Cantrell; I've just been in to see your baby. Let's go down, here, in the hall, where we can sit down and talk a minute."

His expression was cold. I could not tell whether he felt there was any hope for Chris or not. As he followed, I turned and went back down the steps to a bench that was in the hallway.

"Mrs. Grandle," he began, "I can see no hope for your son. It seems to me that hydrocephalus has started to develop; there will probably be urinary problems within a few weeks. I suggest that you find a home somewhere that will take him, and you and your family forget that he was ever born. I will make arrangements for him to be discharged as soon as you wish to leave." With those cold, harsh words, he excused himself, saying that he had other patients to see, and disappeared down the hall.

I couldn't even get up for a few minutes. What would I do? What time was it? To whom would I turn? How could I ever forget this lovely child? I was there, in that cold, strange city, all alone. I did the only thing that I could think of—call Mom. I spotted a pay telephone in a booth nearby.

Yes, Mom could leave right away to come for us. It would be almost five before she got to Baltimore . . . but that didn't matter. I just couldn't spend another night in that terrible little room. I assured her that Chris and I would be watching for her.

I couldn't go back up to Chris's room just yet. I had to get out of that hospital . . . I had to just go somewhere . . . outside. . . . I didn't know where. I started walking—where I went, I don't know. I felt the hot tears rolling down my cheeks. What was I going to do? God, please help me! Please tell me what to do! Where do I turn now for help?

Walking through those lonely streets of that old city, I found an answer forming in my mind. I would take Chris home. . . . Yes, I would put him in a home as Dr. Cantrell had suggested . . . but not the kind that he meant. For as long as God intended for us to have him, Chris would come home to live with his family, where we could care for him and love him.

After I had made up my mind, I found my way to the room where I was staying, packed my small bag, paid my bill to the landlady, and made arrangements for Chris to be discharged, so that we would be ready when Mom arrived.

I was so glad to see her. She had taken time to put a bag of fruit in the car, eliminating our need to stop for food on the return trip home. Chris had drunk a bottle of formula just before he had been discharged, so he was cosy in the car bed and went to sleep shortly after we got on the road.

We were hardly out of Baltimore, before Mom asked the

question that I knew she had wanted to ask from the time I got in the car. "Where are you going to take Chris? Back to Mrs. Henkel's?"

"No, Mom, I'm taking him home!"

"Oh, Judy, do you really think that you should? How are you going to care for him? What is Jimmy going to say? Are you sure that this is the best thing? What about the boys?"

"I know, Mom, I've thought of all of those things. I have been walking the streets of Baltimore since I called you, and I have thought and prayed about it. I can take care of him as well as anybody else . . . maybe better. I'm convinced that his head is no larger than Bob's head. You know all of the men in our family have big heads. They all have trouble getting hats that are large enough. Jimmy will be glad to have Chris at home. He always wants what I want!" And so it went . . . Mom saw that my mind was made up. She promised to do anything that she could to help us . . . and she has more than kept that promise.

It was after eleven when we got home. Everybody was sound asleep. I took Chris, in his car bed, up to our bedroom and put him on the floor at the foot of our bed. I had enough formula for him for one feeding in the morning. . . . The hospital gave me that before we left. Poor baby didn't even have a real bed to sleep in, but it didn't seem to bother him at all. I didn't hear a sound out of him until about six the next morning.

Jimmy sat straight up in bed at the sound of a baby's crying. I calmly told him what the doctor had said, how mad and hurt I was because I did not feel that the doctor could have examined Chris in any way. I told him of my decision to bring Chris home to live with us. Dear Jimmy did not question my decision. His questions were much more practical: What was I going to feed him? Did I have any clothes for him? Where was he going to sleep?

Mom had promised to stay with him while I went to the store for a few necessary things, and Chris could sleep in the car bed a day or so until I could get the bassinet out again.

Shortly before noon, there was a knock at the door. It was delivery men with a beautiful new baby bed. After I got back from the store, Mom had gone downtown and had purchased a new bed for her grandson. She told me later that she felt he was too large for the bassinet. There was just no sense in getting it out of the attic for a week or two.

I had many phone calls to make that day—one was to Dr. Calhoun. I reported to him what had happened, and what I had done. I expected him to tell me that I was wrong, and that I should have taken Dr. Cantrell's advice. Instead, he told me that since the time that Chris was born, he had been studying his medical books and journals to learn all that he could about spina bifida. He felt very frustrated by the fact that almost nothing was written about this condition. He told me that even though he could find nothing in the books to help him, he would always give me all of the help and guidance that he possibly could. We'd just have to work together and do what we could—how much better I felt after talking to him. I somehow felt that I had made the right decision—only time would tell.

I also called Mrs. Henkel, to report that Chris would not be back there . . . at least for the present. He was going to be with his family.

III

The old baby carriage that I had used for the boys came out of Mom's attic. A new dressing table was purchased and set up in the bath downstairs. It was soon evident that we had a baby living at our house.

We didn't go to church that first Sunday that Chris was home, because I was a little fearful of his exposure to some contagious disease. He had not had any of his shots.

Chris was really unhappy when he saw Dr. Calhoun the next week. Something about doctors seemed to frighten him. He screamed at the top of his lungs during the early visits that we made to see Dr. Calhoun.

I made little belly bands out of a lightweight fabric. The doctor said that I should continue to keep his back covered with the sterile dressings, just in case it started to drain again. The regular knit belly bands were hot; besides, they were meant for newborn infants. Chris was growing. The heavy band just did not go around him. There was also the extra area needed to cover the meningocele, which had become less protruding by this time. When he was still at Mrs. Henkel's house, he had begun to roll on his back; he seemed satisfied to lie in that position. It apparently did not cause him any pain.

Bob and Art said that the "bump" on his back reminded them of a telephone dial. Jimmy said that it looked more like a large flower. I could see how either description would fit. I made many of his clothes, because they could not be tight over his back. Most clothing made for infants had elastic around the waist. Those just would not do. Chris needed little shoulder straps on most of his clothes.

By the second Sunday after Chris came home, we were taking him with us whenever we went out, and he went along to church with us that Sunday. He completely won the hearts of the ladies who kept the nursery. They reported to us that he was a good baby, and had a fine time while we were attending the worship service.

Chris was treated as we treated the other children. As we were to tell him later, God made all people different—some with blue eyes, some with brown eyes, some tall, some short—some with good legs, and some with legs that do not work so well. Chris was our son, we were proud of him, and we loved him as much as we loved the older boys.

I continued to keep his shoes on the wrong feet as Mrs. Henkel had done. Dr. Calhoun approved the idea. I also massaged his feet, just as Mrs. Henkel had shown me.

Many times, when I had Chris out walking, people inquired as to whether I was aware that his shoes were on the wrong feet. They seemed a little embarrassed when I explained. Chris was such a beautiful, happy, little fellow that everybody wanted to make a fuss over him. He appeared to be a happy, healthy boy. Few strangers ever noticed that he had any deformities.

After the boys started school, the first of September, Chris and I were alone most of the day. The days were pretty routine . . . caring for a baby of four or five months of age. Chris began to pull himself around in his crib. He rolled over without any trouble. He was even beginning to remain steady when he was propped against a pillow.

Bob and Art spent time talking to him and playing with him whenever they were at home. We could easily see that Chris loved them, and was especially happy when they were around.

One weekend in October, the boys had a school holiday. The family decided that we would travel to Knoxville to visit my brother. After Henry graduated from the University of Virginia in June, he had moved his family to Tennessee, where he was employed at Oak Ridge. We took Chris and Mom with us. Henry lived in a small house at the time, so all of us stayed in a motel. During the day, Chris played and slept in the bed that I had used for Bob and Art, then had loaned to Henry for his children.

Chris was a good traveler; he liked to ride in the car. Staying in a strange place did not bother him at all.

We decided that we would like to have a picture of Chris for our Christmas cards that year. So, in November, when he was six months old, we had a commercial photographer make his portrait. Then he made a group picture of the Grandle brothers that we used as a Christmas gift for the grandmothers, aunts, and uncles.

One evening, shortly before Thanksgiving, Dr. Calhoun called. I could tell by the sound of his voice that he was very excited about something. He started to tell me the story.

He and his wife had taken a few days off to go to Washington. They had registered in a hotel where a conference of physical medicine specialists was being held. His wife wanted to spend one morning shopping, so he decided that he would just stay at the hotel and rest, instead of going with her.

After a while, he wandered down into the lobby and into one of the meeting rooms of the physical medicine conference. He suddenly realized that the speaker was giving a paper on his success with the rehabilitation of spina bifidas.

Dr. Calhoun has said many times during the years since, that he was led into that meeting by a divine power. He had no reason to be there. I, too, feel that God saw to it that Dr. Calhoun heard this one part of the program, prepared for another field of medicine.

"He said that he can even have them walking!" I heard Dr. Calhoun proclaim excitedly at the other end of the wire.

I was almost dumbfounded . . . could I really believe what he was saying? Was there maybe some hope after all? Who is this man? Will he see Chris? When can we get in touch with him?

Dr. Calhoun didn't even let me interrupt; he could guess

the questions that were charging through my mind. He had the name of the doctor, and he would call him the first thing in the morning. He was located in New York. I could see us right then starting out for New York. Mom would take care of the boys. . . . We could go anytime that the doctor would see Chris.

It was late afternoon before he called, but Dr. Calhoun had been able to get in touch with the doctor in New York. Yes, he would see Chris if we really wanted him to, but he felt that we should see a doctor in Richmond, who, he had been assured, could do anything that could be done in New York. The recommendation for us to go to Richmond was given because of the many, many trips to be made for many years to come. Those trips would be much easier for all of us. I was somewhat disappointed, yet what did we have to lose? Dr. Calhoun tried the next day to make the necessary arrangements.

I learned later that the doctor in New York was George C. Deavers. He developed the rehabilitation methods for spina bifidas as a result of what he had learned while treating spinal injuries of the Korean War. He was the only medical doctor at that time to have received the Congressional Medal of Honor. I realized that good comes out of everything . . . even war—as horrible as it is, has some good.

Next evening, when Dr. Calhoun called, he informed me of our appointment to see Dr. Bert Williams at the Medical College of Virginia on January 3.

Christmas that year was very special. By the last of December Chris could fairly well sit up in the chair table that we had gotten for him . . . provided there was a pillow giving him a little support. The boys had great fun trying to get him to unwrap the beautiful, bright packages, especially those that they had so carefully wrapped. Chris seemed to think that they would be much better if he put them in his mouth. Each time his little hand would move in the direction of his mouth with a gift clutched tightly, a bigger hand would grab it and take both little hands, put them on the gift, and demonstrate how to tear the paper. Finally, with much assistance from his big brothers, Chris found each of his gifts. Most of them went straight into his mouth.

Santa had brought the boys additions for their electric trains. They wished to take Chris with them to the basement to watch them set up the trains and then run them. Chris thought that it was much more fun to chew on the rubber deer that had been one of his gifts.

My special gift was one that I shall never forget. About the middle of the day I put Chris on the dressing table to make necessary changes. . . . He was in a very playful mood. Suddenly, I saw his right foot move . . . ever so slightly, but I was sure that it moved. I shouted and hollered for everybody to come see what I had seen. We all stood there watching—Chris thought it was great to get all of that attention. He moved his foot again. We got out the movie camera so that we would be able to show Dr. Calhoun. I was to learn later that this slight movement was the result of the action of a muscle in his abdomen.

The real gift of the holiday season was a belated one. It arrived on January 3. That morning, Jimmy and I got an early start with Chris on the first of a countless number of trips to Richmond. Even though Dr. Calhoun had given us excellent directions for locating Dr. Williams's office at the Medical College of Virginia, we wanted to be sure that we had sufficient time.

The Department of Physical Medicine was located across the street from the main part of the hospital in an older building. Oddly, it reminded me somewhat of the hospital in Baltimore. The memory made me shudder and say a quick prayer that, here, we would find hope instead of despair.

The receptionist said that the doctor would see us shortly, so we sat down in the large lobby, which had a glass-covered model of the Medical College upon a table in the center of the room. Jimmy was nervous. . . . He walked around the model to get various views and to try to keep me from seeing how nervous he was. I felt very much the same way.

After what seemed like hours, we were shown into the doctor's examining room. He asked me to undress Chris so that he might check him thoroughly. The outside office door opened and there stood Dr. Calhoun. He just "happened" to be in Richmond for a medical meeting and thought that he would drop by. I've often wondered about the truth of the story . . . but I was so glad to see him.

Dr. Williams quickly and efficiently completed his examination.

"I'll have him walking before he is two," he said as he looked at me. Then he began to outline what had to be done.

Since the meningocele was not draining, he advised not removing it until there was enough "good" skin on his back to cover it without skin grafting. However, he wanted a plastic surgeon to confirm his recommendations. He wanted us to go by to see the surgeon that day. He prescribed a program of physical therapy to straighten Chris's legs and increase the range of motion in both of his hips and his knees. Dr. Calhoun told him that our local hospital had a physical therapist and that there would soon be one working with cerebral palsied children who probably could see Chris. Finally, Dr. Williams wanted to see Chris again in six weeks.

I was dazed . . . I kept saying over and over to Jimmy . . . walking by the time he is two. I just couldn't believe it. I would be so glad if he could ever walk . . . but before he was two!

The plastic surgeon agreed with Dr. Williams. We should probably wait a year or more before trying to repair the back, since there did not seem to be any immediate reason for the surgery. He wanted to check Chris about every other time that he was seen by Dr. Williams.

Dr. Calhoun made all of the arrangements for Chris to be treated by the physical therapist at our hospital five days a week. I was to give him exercises at home three times a day.

Chris's legs lay out to the sides. Both hips were dislocated and very tight. His knees were stiff and were bent at about a ninety-degree angle, which meant that when he was lying on his back, the bottoms of his feet almost touched. The position of his legs, and the fact that he was a breech birth, caused both of his legs to be broken at birth. It was probably these broken bones, which had gone undetected for several days, that caused the high fever which he carried during the first several weeks of his life.

The treatment given consisted of massaging, stretching, and pulling of his legs into a more natural position. I'm sure that if he had had any feeling in his legs and feet, the pain would have been unbearable. Since there were no nerves in his legs or feet, he enjoyed the attention and somebody's talking to him. This did keep me rather busy, but I managed.

After about a month of treatments from the PT at the hospital, Dr. Calhoun made arrangements for the new PT at the Cerebral Palsy Clinic to begin seeing Chris. I had mixed feelings about taking Chris to this clinic. I didn't want anybody to think that my son had cerebral palsy. To be quite honest about it, at first I did not know much about the condition. Chris was seen by appointment so, at first, I did not see many of the other patients at the clinic.

Dr. Williams was pleased with the progress that was made in those first six weeks of treatment. The range of motion in the knees and legs had improved greatly. He instructed the PT to continue the stretching, and to add exercises that would develop Chris's hands and arms. The doctor wanted sufficient strength in Chris's upper torso for walking on crutches when the time came.

Chris was pulling himself around on the floor with his arms and was soon able to get himself into a sitting position. The PT suggested that we should get a set of wooden blocks that he could push down on the floor as he sat and then lift himself to a new position. Well, that didn't work at all. Getting a child of ten to twelve months of age to understand lifts was more than we could manage. Chris enjoyed the fun of throwing the blocks around with his other toys and was quite content to get about on my hardwood floors by the pushing-and-sliding method.

Gerry agreed to come back that next spring to help me clean the house. While she was there, I was exposed to mumps. She promised that she would come back to take care of Chris and my family if I got the mumps.

Sure enough, one morning, several weeks later, I awoke and felt a soreness in my neck and throat . . . I had an outstanding case of the mumps! Jimmy went for Gerry, and she was there in time to get breakfast for the children. I was quite ill for a few days. After I felt somewhat better, Chris wanted to be on my bed to play. He was exposed to the mumps, I'm sure, but he never got them. Since then, I have learned of the dangers of exposing him to mumps because of the weakness of his urinary system. Again, God was looking after him.

The doctors had told us that Chris would probably not be able to develop any control over either his bladder or his bowels. I remember how the urine sometimes did not seem to have any force behind it as it came from his penis. One day, I was so delighted because there was enough pressure for him to "christen" the wall as I was changing his diaper. I told some of my friends that I did not even want to wash the wall. That was just one small triumph for Chris. Dr. Williams told me that he thought it would be possible to train him with a time schedule after he grew older. At this early age, he normally passed a very constipated stool. Sometimes, he would need to be aided with a massaging in his lower back to help pass these stools, which the family referred to as "Chrissie's marbles."

Chris became my automatic cleaner. He liked to be on the floor most of the time. Sometimes, he would pull or push himself as he lay on his stomach. At other times, he would sit up and push himself around on his bottom. Most of the time his little feet would be crossed in front of him, the result of the movement that he made as he rolled from his stomach to the sitting position. Toys were always underfoot. Chris's little overalls usually looked like scrub rags, but he was happy.

Even at this early age, he began to learn that he could get a big brother down to his size by grabbing a leg and just hanging on. He was developing strength in his arms, even if he didn't use the blocks as the PT suggested.

After the first month or so of taking Chris to the clinic for treatments, the PT suggested that I attend the meetings of the parents' group. I had a great many excuses. I could see no reason for my meeting with these people that I didn't know. How could we possibly have anything in common? I had other things that I wanted to do with my spare time . . . what little bit I had.

Before Chris was born, I had become involved in PTA work at both the local and state levels. I continued to do as much in that organization as I could. Mom would take care of the boys when I needed to be out of town overnight. I also taught a class of primary children and sang in the church choir. . . . I went back to that soon after Chris was born. I enjoyed membership in a local garden club and meeting with sorority sisters twice a month. Dr. Williams had told me on one of the first visits that I should be involved in activities outside of my home and not devote my every waking hour to Chris. I assured him that I did not think he needed to worry about that. Sometimes, through the years, I've wondered if maybe I took him too literally, for I have been involved in many church and community activities during the years.

Jimmy's brother was the treasurer of the Cerebral Palsy Clinic Board. He talked to me sometimes about the people whose children were being treated there. He thought that it might be good for me to get to know some of them. The Board had been able to add a speech motivationist to the clinic staff, and one of my sorority friends brought her mentally retarded son in for sessions. I learned that she attended the meetings of the parents' group. I finally agreed to attend one meeting.

I went to the meeting thinking that I would sit back and just listen . . . but I never could keep quiet. I found myself involved in the conversation. Here were parents facing problems similar to some that we faced. One, I remember so well. How do you discipline a small child who has no feeling in his little bottom? One parent told me that she had very good results by isolating her son in his bedroom until he could change his behavior so that it was acceptable to the family.

We tried the isolation and it worked. Believe me, we faced all of the problems of discipline that one faces with any happy little boy who has a quick mind and older brothers who had, by now, found out that a little teasing did not hurt their brother.

I found that the meetings with these parents of cerebral palsied children were very helpful to me, and that sometimes I had found a method that would help someone else. I learned to know most of the cerebral palsy patients at the clinic—each had a slightly different problem or muscular involvement. I learned to love these spastic children and to no longer see them as some weird mass of humanity to be avoided.

There were other patients at the center besides CP's, however. One little boy, a year or so older than Chris, had had polio. A girl had suffered paralysis in one side of her body as a result of an accident, and there were several retarded children who came in only for speech work. They were all children with special problems, and the clinic was trying to meet as many of these needs as possible. Little was I to know, then, that my family and I would become very involved in working with these children and their families to develop a program that would help each of them in their development.

The program of therapy at the center seemed to work well for Chris. Dr. Williams was pleased with the progress that he was making. During Chris's first year and a half, we made a visit to Richmond every six weeks, and every other visit we also saw the plastic surgeon. In the fall, both Dr. Williams and Dr. Hunter, the plastic surgeon, felt that the time was approaching when Chris should undergo the surgery to repair his back. So, arrangements were made for him to be admitted to the Medical College of Virginia Hopsital in the early part of November.

Dr. Williams told us that he had selected Dr. Hunter as the surgeon because of his work with spinal cord injuries of men injured in the Korean War. Dr. Hunter expected to call in a neurosurgeon during the surgery to determine if there would be any chance of restoring use to Chris's legs.

They recommended that I plan to stay in Richmond during the time that Chris would be hospitalized.

IV

Our family's plans for the operation developed: Mom would look after Bob and Art; I would stay at the home of my college roommate who lived in nearby Bon Air; and Jimmy would remain in Richmond until after the surgery was over, probably the first day or so. Dr. Hunter advised us to have nurses or someone with Chris around the clock. It was absolutely essential that Chris lie on his stomach for three weeks following the surgery. He explained the danger of infection to us because of the open spinal column. The operation was a hazardous one, but necessary.

After the admitting routine, we were taken to a ninth-floor room, blocked into eight little cubicles and furnished with eight little white, iron baby beds. Beside each bed, in each cubicle, was a white bedside cabinet and a single, white, straight chair. The walls and the partitions were painted a light shade of green. The top of each partition was glass with imbedded wire. If a child were able to stand up in the crib, it could see other children in the room. The glass also made the room on the northeast side of the building much lighter. During the two weeks that Chris lay in the first bed inside the door, I memorized every inch of that room.

Shortly after the nurse got Chris settled in his bed, the interns and residents started to arrive to look at this new creature who had just been admitted. They fired questions at both Jimmy and me as they looked Chris over.

They seemed amazed when we told them that he was able to sit up alone. They were sure that he needed support.

Finally, Jimmy offered to have Chris show them. So, they took Chris out in the hall where there was a table. Chris was placed on the edge of the table in a sitting position. He sat up as big as life and began talking to the doctors. They could not believe what they were seeing or hearing. Chris had been less than a year old when he began to put two and three words together. Now, by the time the he was eighteen months old, the sentences were more advanced. He had long-ago gotten over his fear of doctors. He loved to talk to anybody who would listen.

A shortage of nurses existed, then, as now. The first night, we were able to get a practical nurse to come on the first shift, but there was no one to come on the late shift. One of the floor nurses volunteered to come back. She said that the next day was her day off, and she did not mind to help us out in that way. I agreed to take the day shift.

Chris was taken to surgery early the next morning. Dr. Hunter told us that it would probably take several hours, maybe four or five . . . but Jimmy and I did not leave the hospital. We waited anxiously, and prayed that the operation would be successful. Finally, Dr. Hunter appeared in his green operating-room clothes. He was smiling as he approached. Our spirits rose!

Chris had come through the operation in fine shape. Dr. Hunter was afraid that they had been unable to generate any use in his legs. There were more than sixty-five stitches in his back. Dr. Hunter grinned, "You can call him 'Stinky' . . . the scar will be in the shape of a big S on his back."

He explained how he had cut away all of the molelike skin covering the meningocele, and then pulled two overlapping flaps of skin together. This skin, covering muscle tissue, he had used to cover and protect the opening in the spinal column. He had simply pushed the bundle of nerves back into the spinal column before covering it.

Late in the afternoon, the orderlies brought Chris back to the room. He lay there, so still and quiet, with tubes running out of him everywhere. It was frightening; this was the first time in my life that I had been around anyone who had had major surgery. After calling home to Mom and the boys, to let them know that the operation had gone all right, we drove out to rest with my friend in Bon Air.

The night was long, for I had difficulty sleeping. I think Jimmy, too, was awake several times during the night. We were up before the alarm sounded at five-thirty. I had to be at the hospital before the nurse left at seven, and the ten-mile drive into the city might be slow through heavy early morning traffic.

After checking that Chris had come safely through the night, Jimmy headed for home, and I sat on that straight white chair by Chris's bed to keep watch over him. He could not roll over, and he was very unhappy when he was tied down. The first several days he was rather quiet and seemed to sleep frequently. How do you feed a small child who is lying on his stomach? At first they gave him milk, which he only half-way took from the bottle because he had learned to drink from a cup. He had not yet fully mastered the use of a straw. As the days went by, the doctor returned him to a regular diet.

Finding his fingers much more useful than silverware, he raised his head up, turtle fashion, to eat. He much preferred to feed himself. The menus made little difference; he still used his fingers. He was the center of attraction at mealtime—the dietician and all of the nurses gathered to watch. Tomato soup and chocolate puddings made fine eating. Surprisingly, Chris made little mess.

Each day I got up at five-thirty and drove to the hospital to relieve the night nurse. We finally found a black practical nurse who took the night shift. She was wonderful. We also had to find another nurse for the first evening shift. The first practical nurse we had went to sleep on the job, and the floor supervisor caught her.

Soon, we became friends with the parents of the other children who moved in and out of the room's seven other beds. One little girl, who had surgery on a cleft lip, lived not far from our hometown, Harrisonburg. Her mother and

I enjoyed each other's company as we cared for our children.

Most of the children placed in our room were there for only a few days: some tonsillectomies, some plastic surgery, and some general surgery cases. I was truly amazed at the wonders of plastic surgery that I saw while I was there. More than ever, I realized that Chris was not the only imperfect child in the world. All of God's angels are created differently. No two are cut from the same pattern.

As Chris's body began to heal, and some of the tubes were removed, the nurses suggested that I wheel his bed down the hall to the playroom, where movies were shown and where there were other children who played with Chris, who enjoyed these recreation periods.

During the second weekend that Chris was in the hospital, Mom and Jimmy brought the boys to Richmond to see me. Some of our high school friends lived in Richmond, and they took all of us to see the "Ice Capades." It was a great show, and helped all of us to relax. I especially enjoyed getting away from the hospital routine and the sitting by Chris's bedside. Watching that he did not turn over was hard, exhausting work. Each evening as I went home to Bon Air, I appreciated the nurses who took the other two shifts.

On the Monday before Thanksgiving, Dr. Hunter removed all of the stitches in Chris's back and indicated that he might let us go home for the holiday. Excitedly, I called Jimmy to ask him to come and to help us to come home. He had ridden the bus to Richmond the first weekend, and I thought that he would do that again, even though he was thoroughly disgusted with the schedule. It had taken him about eight hours by bus to make the two-and-a-half-hour automobile trip.

I was shocked to find Jimmy beside Chris's bed when I arrived to take my shift on Wednesday morning. I knew that the bus was not due to arrive until midafternoon. He grinned rather sheepishly and admitted that he had hitchhiked to Richmond. He had been lucky and gotten a ride on a truck. Most of the night he had been on the hard, straight chair by Chris's bed.

Chris was released that day, and we were home for Thanksgiving. We had so much for which to give thanks! Dr. Hunter suggested that I tie Chris in bed so that he would not turn over during the night for the first week. It made him unhappy, so I propped pillows beside him to prevent his turning. Oddly, he seemed to know that he was not supposed to lie on his back. Yet, on that twenty-first day, the day that Dr. Hunter said he might turn, he began to roll over without anyone showing him that he could. He just seemed to know that his back had healed enough for him to begin lying on it once again.

Just before Christmas, we made another trip to Richmond to see both Dr. Williams and Dr. Hunter. The incision had healed nicely, and now it was time for Chris to have his first braces. Dr. Williams called the brace maker and explained exactly what to do, but he also wrote a prescription for us to carry down the street to the brace shop. The doctor gave us directions to the small shop on the hill below the hospital. In an old building that looked as though it might not last much longer, there was a small fitting room partitioned off in one corner. Further back in the shop, was a variety of metal-working machines—machinery much like that which I had seen in the shoe repair shop at home. I noticed pieces of leather and scraps of metal lying about on the floor. An older gentleman greeted us. He wore a green eye-shade and celluloid cuffs over his shirt. I assumed he was the bookkeeper, for he called a younger man from the back and gave him the prescription. The old gentleman chatted with Chris and gave him a sucker before we left.

The young man called Tommy, whom we have depended on for over twenty years, gently placed Chris on the table in the fitting room. Under him lay a large piece of brown wrapping paper. Tommy took a pencil and began the process of measuring Chris for his first pair of braces by outlining his body and legs on the paper. Then came the tape measure that Tommy wore around his neck as though he were a tailor. He took measurements at many points and recorded them on the paper under Chris. Tommy told us that we would have to go up town to purchase the shoes required for the braces; then we could drop them off at the shop before we left for home. He estimated that the braces would be ready in six to eight weeks. When ready, he would call to make an appointment to have them fitted. Dr. Williams also had to approve the braces.

Home again, to wait for the call and celebrate the Christmas holidays!

V

It was almost the last of January before we heard that the braces were finally ready. I thought I knew a lot about braces. My aunt, a polio victim who I had visited a great deal when I was young, had worn a brace on one leg. However, I didn't expect what I saw when Tommy came out of the shop carrying Chris's braces. He brought two little leg braces that were attached to something called a knight brace. I can imagine it got that name because it looked as though it could have served some knight of ancient days as a suit of armor. A metal frame fit under his arms and extended around the back. His body, from his armpits to his hips, was enclosed in this frame. Across the front was a heavy canvas pad fastened on each side with a series of belts and buckles. At the end of each leg was a little white shoe.

In the fitting room, Tommy lay the braces on the table, where weeks before, he had placed the brown wrapping paper. He gently lay a screaming Chris into the braces and began to fasten the array of belts and buckles. He carefully checked the fit of the braces before he stood Chris up and asked that I support him so other checks could be made. Chris didn't want any part of those things; he continued to scream and reached out, trying his very best to grab hold of me. I fought to keep back my own tears and the temptation to hold him close in my arms so he would know he was safe.

One of my first questions was, "How in the world will I change his diapers?" Tommy informed me that I would have to take his braces off each time. He gave instructions about

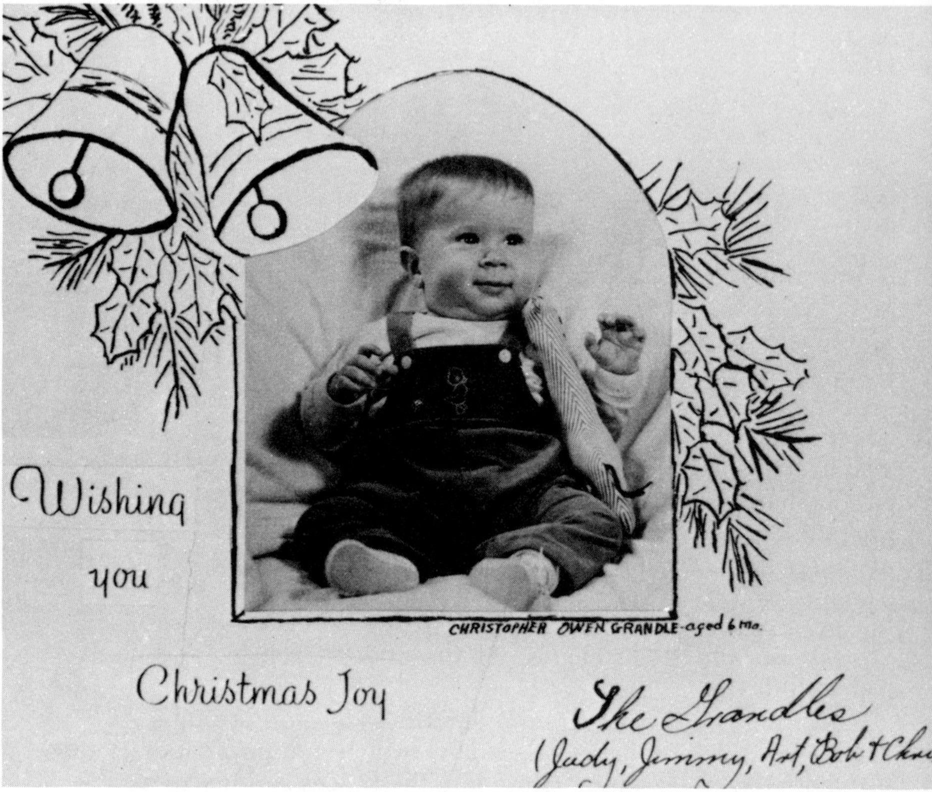
Wishing
you
Christmas Joy
CHRISTOPHER OWEN GRANDLE-aged 6 mo.
The Grandles
(Judy, Jimmy, Art, Bob +

We were proud to send this picture of Chris to our friends that first Christmas that he was with us.

waxing the leather to keep it soft and nonirritating to his skin. Then, we took the braces off, to go up the street to see Dr. Williams; Chris was so very unhappy and so very vocal about it. People on the street might have thought we were abusing the child.

Dr. Williams asked me to put Chris back in the braces. Even though he helped, it took almost a half-hour. Again, Chris turned on the screaming. The doctor checked the braces carefully before he announced that they seemed to fit very well. "Start putting them on for an hour in the morning and an hour in the afternoon; then increase the time some each day, until he is in them most of the time. Watch his skin very carefully for red spots that indicate the brace is not fitting properly." Since there is no feeling, I had to be especially careful about pressure sores developing. Chris's lack of nerves and poor circulation would make sores difficult to heal. Dr. Williams wanted Chris standing while he was in his braces, so he instructed Jimmy to build a "standing table" (I thought all tables stood). Dr. Williams drew a sketch and told us that the physical therapist would be able to give more detailed information. Also, he wanted Chris to again see the physical therapist twice a week. A long prescription was written for the physical therapist to follow. And so began the tear-filled process of teaching Chris to walk.

At home, I put Chris in his braces and placed him on the floor, thinking that he might pull himself around a little. He just lay there screaming, big tears running down his cheeks. I could hardly stand it, but I knew that somehow or other I had to get him to the point where he would accept the imprisonment of his body in this frame of metal and leather. I let him yell!

Jimmy got the standing table built. It was very much like his feeding table, except without a seat. By the second day, I was able to put him into the table, instead of laying him on the floor as I had done the first day. There were still tears, but not so many. Even those few soon stopped when I was able to get him interested in playing with the toys that I put on the table.

Hey! This wasn't so bad after all! It was play time. I had won the first battle!

Chris was soon wearing his brace several hours each morning and afternoon, without any indications of a pressure sore starting. Harry, the physical therapist, told me how to have Jimmy build a set of parallel bars. Jimmy, who is very capable in building or repair, constructed the bars so that they were adjustable. Harry said the bars should be at a height that would enable Chris to rest his forearm on the bar when he stood between them. Knowing that Chris would grow, Jimmy had constructed the bars so that they could be adjusted to almost any height.

After ten days or so of just standing in his standing table, Chris was moved to the parallel bars. It was tear time again. The poor little child was so frightened that he just stood between the bars, gripping each one and shaking. He was supposed to pull himself along through the bars. How did I make him understand? Words didn't work! He was just plain frightened! We'd try again in the afternoon, when Bob and Art were there.

Bob and Art tried to help me work with him. They were on the floor making faces, to entertain him and to get him to stop crying. Both of them got in the bars in front of him and kneeled to pull themselves through the bars, hoping that he would follow them. No luck.

What could we do? Finally, the boys hit upon the idea of slowly pulling the bars along the floor. We tried it. Chris pulled his little body a few inches, to keep himself in a vertical position. We tried it again; again he moved a few inches—again and again. He was beginning to get the idea, but he never released that grip he had on the bars.

Next problem—how did we get him to move his hands along the bars? A good question! We tried everything we could think of.

One day, a senior citizen living across the street dropped in when Chris was standing in his bars, and we were trying unsuccessfully to get him to move. The neighbor stood at the far end of the bars and held out a bright, shiny roll of candy. Chris's face lit up; he let go of the bar with one hand to reach for the candy. Suddenly, I got the idea that maybe we could bribe him. I took the candy and held it just out of his reach. It worked!!! Chris pulled his little stiff body several inches. I was mean . . . I moved the candy. His little hands moved on the bars, and again he pulled his little body toward the candy. Everybody cheered! Chris laughed and got the candy.

We must have used hundreds of those candies in our efforts to get Chris to learn to walk in his parallel bars. After he discovered he could do something new, he became a show-off. He demonstrated his new skill for anybody who came around.

Both Dr. Williams and Harry were amazed at how quickly he had learned to pull himself through the parallel bars. Bob and Art were a tremendous help in reaching this first goal. They worked with him for hours at a time. I found that I had very little time with housekeeping chores and keeping Chris socially acceptable. Every time that Chris needed a diaper change, it was necessary to remove his braces completely. The process took a half-hour. I couldn't help but laugh. Sometimes, just about the time that I got the last buckle fastened on the brace, he needed another change. I couldn't win. Fortunately, I had found a silicone preparation that seemed to give his skin the necessary protection; without feeling, he suffered no discomfort.

Shortly after Chris began to feel comfortable in his parallel bars, Harry began a program to teach him to fall. He explained to me that for Chris's safety, he needed to learn to relax when he fell. This training attempted to help him overcome some of the fear he had of falling.

After several weeks with the bars at elbow height, Harry said to lower them to hand height. More tears! but with the aide of the boys, and the rolls of candy, Chris was soon pulling himself along between the bars. He learned to turn around when he got to the end and go back the other way. So, back and forth he went. So, at about twenty-two months of age, he was ready to be fitted with crutches.

In less than eight weeks since we saw Tommy to get his braces, he was back to get crutches! He was not unhappy at seeing Tommy. Dr. Williams prescribed Everett's canes, explaining to us that these would make Chris bear weight on his hands rather than on his armpits. Such pressure on the nerves in the armpits over many years causes paralysis in the arms.

The metal Everett's canes extended several inches above the elbows. The hand grips slanted toward the front, making a difference between the one used on the right and left side.

How well I remember the first time that I gave the crutches to Chris! We all expected that he would take the crutches and start walking across the floor. He had progressed to the point where he went from one end of the parallel bars to the other, then turned and went back. He repeated the process time and again, without anybody telling him to do it. I expected, replacing the parallel bars, the same thing to happen with the crutches.

I put him in the kitchen in front of the refrigerator, where all the family could watch as I put the tiny little crutches on his arms. He began to scream and shed those big tears when I placed his hands on the hand grips. I released him and moved back across the room so that he could walk toward me. . . . I had a roll of candies in my hand. He was so frightened. As he shook, those big tears fell on the floor. Nothing that I could do or say calmed him. I was so disappointed that I felt like crying too. I took him in my arms, loved him, and vowed we'd try again tomorrow. Maybe Harry could help us.

Harry had no more luck than we did. After more tears and more trembling, I finally realized that we were asking this small child to do something that he had never seen performed. I recalled that Bob and Art had gotten on their knees and pulled themselves along in the parallel bars to show him the way. Chris did not understand what to do with these pieces of metal on his arms. I wondered what would happen if all of the family were to walk on crutches for a while.

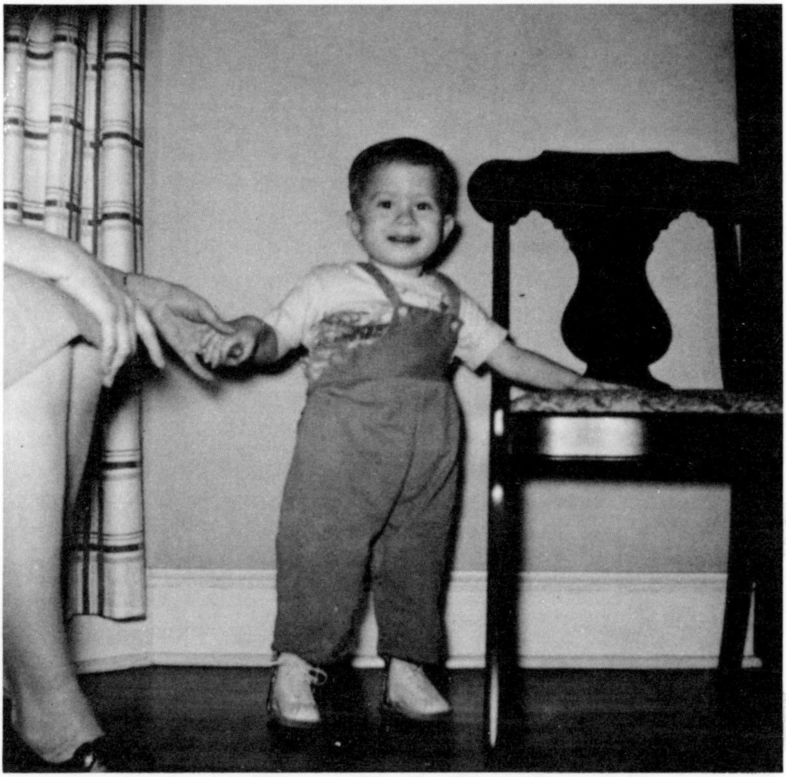

Chairs and mother's hand helped to teach Chris how to stand with his new braces.

Harry agreed that might help. He had never tried to teach a child less than two years old to walk on crutches; he didn't know any more about it than I did. He thought that he could round up four pairs of old crutches to lend us. That day, I went home from the center, armed with four pairs of crutches. Jimmy and the boys were not sure about the idea, but they were willing to do anything that might help Chris. All of us began to walk on the crutches whenever we were in the house. We put Chris's crutches out of sight for a few days. He was the only one who didn't have those pieces of metal on his arms.

Several days later, we decided to try the crutches again. This time, Jimmy, Bob, and Art stood on their crutches, as I sat on the floor in front of Chris. He had no tears this time, just an expression on his face that showed he still wasn't sure that he could do what Bob and Art were doing. After a little persuasion, a promise of candy, and more demonstrations by the boys and Jimmy, he took his first step! We all were so excited that we almost scared him. He took another little step and then another. We were jubilant! Chris was walking. . . . Dr. Williams's promise was a reality!!! Chris was walking before he was two years old. He was only twenty-three months old at the time. The family continued to use the crutches for a short while, but as Chris became more confident, we used them less and less. Finally, they were returned to the center for use by someone else.

Harry concentrated more and more on the technique of falling. He taught Chris how to throw his crutches out of the way so that he would not get an arm caught when he fell. We knew the danger of other injuries from falling on a crutch. Chris also worked on learning the techniques of getting up. This meant that he had to unlock the hip joints, get himself to a standing position by using his crutches, and relock his braces. It was not an easy task for anybody, much less a guy that was only a little over two years old. He learned to do it!

At first, his gate was only what is called a "four-point" gate. He put his crutches out in front of him and then slid his

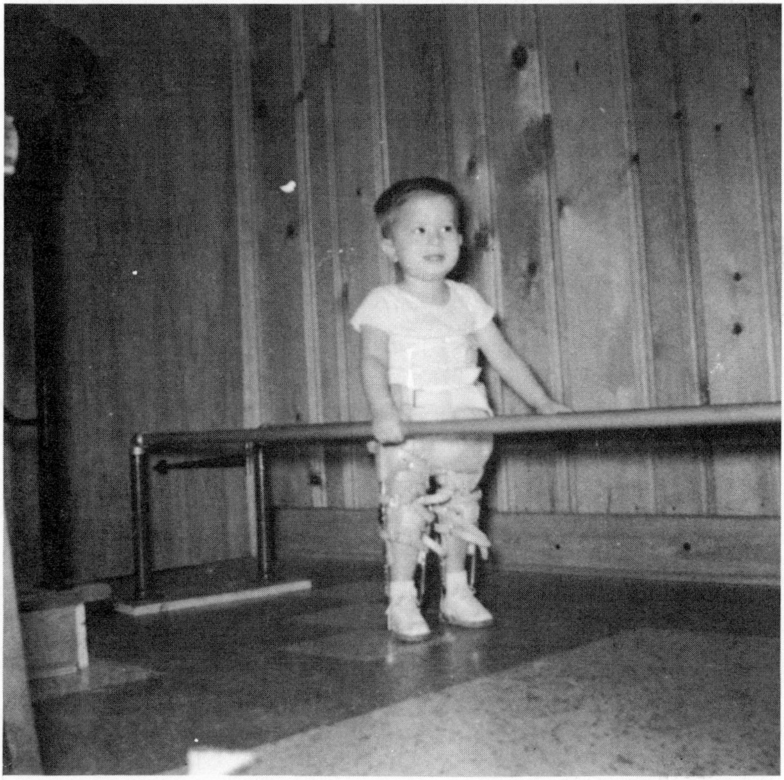

There were so many buckles on those first braces. Sometimes Chris didn't get completely dressed to try out the parallel bars.

feet forward. Repeating the process over and over, slowly, Chris got there. He practiced walking during the summer on the sidewalk in front of our house. He was so tiny. . . . Motorists would stare as they went by; I was so proud of him that I wanted the world to see how well he could do.

Each day that Chris lived, and each new thing he learned to do, was a gift from God—a new joy for all of our family. Often, people have expressed sympathy or sadness because we have what they call an "afflicted child." I used to get almost angry at such people, but I realize now that they have never understood God's making all of His children different. He has allowed us to have one of the very special children. I think I realized this gift more and more as I met with the parents of the children who were treated at the center. Many of them were bitter and frustrated because their child had appeared normal at birth, but something happened which shattered many of the hopes and dreams they held for that child. They were not willing to accept the fact that God had a design, one, sometimes, different from our own plan.

Even though, at two years of age, Chris was walking on his crutches, we continued to have him work in his parallel bars. He learned to lift himself from the floor and swing through. He had hours of fun, playing on the front porch on the bars. It looked as if he was always trying something new, just to show off. One day, I noticed that he seemed to be stomping his right foot. The next time we went to the center, I excitedly reported this behavior to Harry. He almost called me a liar. It was, he said, impossible for Chris to do that. Chris was braced in such a manner that he could not possibly raise one foot independently of the other. Harry said, "Let's put him in the bars, here, at the center and watch." Naturally, Chris just walked up and down in the way that he had been doing the last time he saw Harry. I was so mad. How was I going to prove that I was right? I finally decided that the movie camera was the answer. I took a film of Chris stomping that right foot. Dr. Williams and Harry finally had to believe

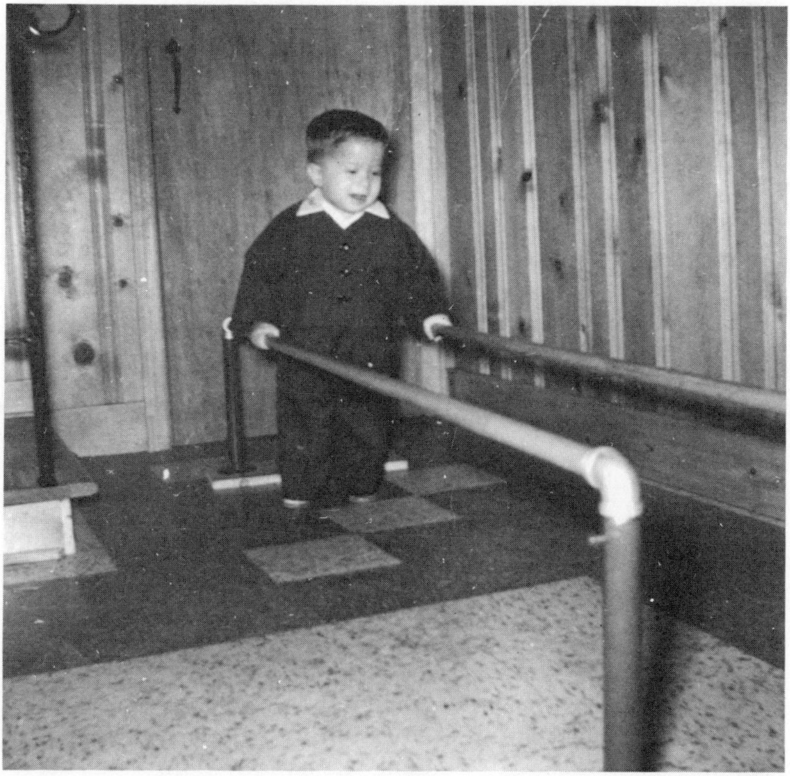

All dressed up and no place to go. The parallel bars did become a "fun" place to walk before Chris tried to walk on crutches.

me. I was sure that Chris was gaining control of his legs, but Dr. Williams felt that Chris was using one of his abdominal muscles to generate this movement.

We continued to make the frequent trips to Richmond. Tommy had to adjust the braces and the crutches as Chris grew. Dr. Williams checked his progress and carefully watched his development. Dr. Calhoun, whom the boys started calling "Uncle Charley," was always at the other end of the phone when I needed him.

The parents elected me their representative to the center board to serve with Dr. Calhoun, the newly elected chairman of the board. We were constantly working to provide sufficient financing for the center. The program was growing, and a part-time teacher had been added to the staff to provide academic work for those children who could not attend public schools. Sometimes, I became frustrated by the red tape that some of the patients had to go through to secure required braces through the State Crippled Children's Bureau. The child was measured for a brace, but it arrived six to ten months later. Naturally it didn't fit; the child was grown. Then, there was another delay while the brace was altered. Fortunately, we were able to provide the bracing that Chris required, and did not experience such delays. The inefficient process of obtaining braces was really a waste of taxpayers' money, and it was one of the things that the parents' group tried to correct. The situation did improve.

During the summers before Chris's birth, Jimmy, the boys, and I had shared an apartment at the beach with the families of friends. We had gone the summer Chris was born, for a few days late in July, but we skipped the next summer because I was afraid that sand would get in his back. The first summer he was braced, we were back at the beach. Four families rented a four-apartment building. Each family had its own apartment. Because of Chris, we decided to occupy one of the downstairs apartments.

Chris had as much fun as the rest of the gang. He loved to sit and play in the sand, just at the edge of the water. As

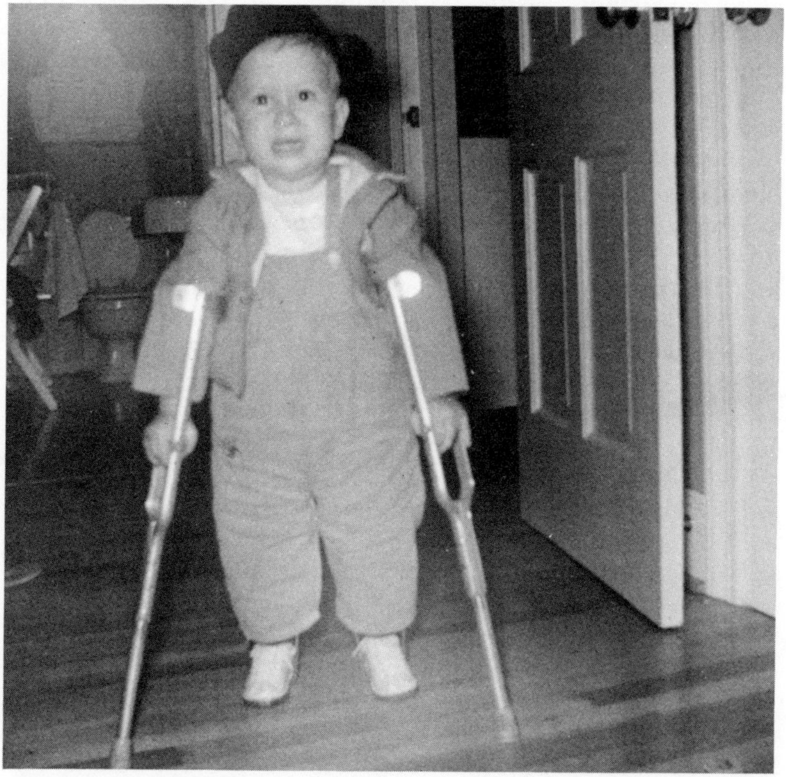

Those first crutches were really scary and caused all of us a lot of tears.

the waves came in with the tide, he scooted backwards on his little bottom. Sometimes, the waves turned him over. He didn't mind at all. He'd just come up spitting and go back for more.

One evening, without thinking, I let him get down on the floor of the apartment without his shoes. He had a great time playing and scooting about the apartment. When I picked him up, I discovered that he had rubbed a "strawberry" on each foot. I was upset, for I knew his feet did not heal very well. I remembered that Uncle Charley had used rather strong language when he saw that an incision had been made in the side of Chris's foot during his surgery, apparently to give a blood transfusion. The incision had healed, but the process had been slow. Luckily that was the next to the last day we were at the beach, so I got in touch with Uncle Charley as soon as we got home. He recommended that I keep the sores open as much as possible and expose them to the heat rays of an ordinary light bulb. I used a photo shade for the light bulb.

That healing process was most interesting to observe. It was slow, but the sores healed around the edges toward the center. Each day the sores were slightly smaller. The one on the right foot healed first. It had been smaller. The left foot was almost healed up in about four weeks. After we had been out to a party one night, I decided I would put the light on Chris's foot while I got ready for bed. During the evening, I had consumed at least five cups of coffee, so I felt wide awake as I lay on the bed. Jimmy asked me about the light on Chris's foot. "I'll turn it off in a minute. With all of that coffee it will be hours before I can sleep," I remember saying as I awakened to find the sun shining in my eyes.

I jumped out of bed and ran over to the baby bed where Chris was lying, still asleep. I was horrified by the sight that I saw; the still-burning light had scorched a circle on the sheet of the bed. Where Chris had had a tiny, almost healed sore, there was now a large, black-looking blister, the size of a silver dollar. Sometime during the night Chris had evidently rolled over so that his foot lay against that hot light bulb. I felt so stupid and upset as I called Uncle Charley out of bed. How could anyone be so unthinking as to do something that foolish? I should have know better. But what was done was done; now we had to deal with it. How was I going to get Chris in his braces? Dr. Williams insisted that he wear them most of the day. Uncle Charley said we should be very, very careful not to break the blister. He suggested that I make a circle of cotton around it for protection. The blister extended about a half-inch above the surface of his foot. No shoe would ever go over the blister and Chris could not wear the braces without a shoe. It has often been said that necessity is the mother of invention, and so it seemed.

I went down to the local shoe repair shop and explained my problem. Together, we worked out a way that he would make a sole to fit in the brace. Then I could use a strap around the ankle to keep his foot in place. It worked! The brace looked very odd, but Chris thought it was great. He enjoyed pointing out the fact that his mother had burnt his foot and that he had a pretty bandage sticking out. I'm sure people wondered what kind of a mother the child had. It was late August when the accident occured, but it was almost Christmas before we could put his shoe back on his foot.

Being a boy, Chris learned to take up for himself when he was playing with his brothers. At a very early age he learned that crutches could be used for things other than walking. A crutch quickly put between the legs of a passing human would bring the person down to where Chris could use his arms on a pretty equal basis. I was often amused when my friends brought their children to play with Chris. They always cautioned the children to be careful and not to hurt Chris; I would in turn caution the children not to let Chris hurt them. Chris was used to roughhousing with the older boys, who could take more than children the age of Chris. He had discovered that a crutch could be used as a club and that he could reach much farther than an unarmed opponent.

At times, Chris was a devilish little guy. He always liked

to tease and do things to get the boys to play with him. They began to call him "Stink-pot," a variation of Dr. Hunter's suggested "Stinky." Sometimes this name of Stink-pot was shortened to "Pot" or "Pottie." It was a name the family continued to use for many years. Even Mother often inquired about Pottie. Sometimes I explained to strangers that we had this child to spoil and we did a pretty good job with the spoiling.

During one period, before Chris was operated on the first time, he seemed to know when Jimmy and I were going out or when the family was going somewhere in the evening, and he could not be included. Thinking he was all settled in bed, being just about ready to leave the house, I heard him make a little crying sound. Then I heard the sound of him being sick. He seemed to have the skill, if you want to call it that, of vomiting at will. Naturally, we were delayed. The first time or two it happened, I was concerned, but knowing that Gerry was there to care for him, I just changed his bed and night clothes and went on. It happened several times, but after checking with Uncle Charley to make sure that he was not really sick, we did not make much fuss over it. We routinely cleaned him up, put him back to bed, and went on with our plans. He soon stopped using this maneuver to keep us at home.

Shortly after Chris began walking on crutches, I found plastic pants that opened on the sides and held either a folded diaper or a disposable pad in the center. The side opening made it possible for me to change Chris without removing the braces. This new tremendous time-saver also made it easier for other people to take care of him.

He stayed with Gerry in her new home near town, when he was just three, while Jimmy and I were gone on a four-week trip to California with Jimmy's boss and his wife. The boys spent part of the time with my brother and then came back to spend the last two weeks at home. Gerry and her new husband moved into our home for those two weeks. Several times before we had been away for short trips, Gerry and her husband had taken care of our boys.

Life at our house had developed into pretty much a routine of a young mother with three boys who was involved in church and community affairs. I employed an amazing black woman about the age of my mother to come in one day a week to help with the cleaning. Even though she was totally deaf, she always knew everything that was happening in town. She had learned to read lips and seemed to be able to understand women quite well. But she had difficulty in understanding men. She loved Chris and he loved her. There was no communication problem at all. She would often look after him when I needed to be away from the house for several hours.

I was convinced that Chris would grow into manhood, able to do anything any other person could do, if he wanted. He had to do it in his own special way, but he would do it.

Each Christmas, for many years, we had taken the boys too see a very special Santa Claus in a department store in Richmond. They would always sit on his knee and have their pictures taken. Chris, too, had to go to see Santa. That first Christmas after he began to walk at twenty-three months, Chris walked up to Santa. Santa didn't know how to pick him up; he tried, then finally gave it up as hopeless, for the braces made Chris rigid from top to bottom. However, Chris stood beside Santa's knee to have his picture taken and to tell him what he wanted for Christmas.

VI

Chris continued to go several times a week to see Harry, the physical therapist. Dr. Williams felt that Chris's back was now strong enough to remove the "knight" brace and leave only long leg braces joined with a band that went around his body below his waist. The new bracing gave him much more freedom of movement. Chris soon developed the ability to lift himself and swing back and forth in his parallel bars. Also, it was now time for him to learn a "swing-through" gait on his crutches. This skill would add speed to his walking and make it possible for him to walk about as fast as most people walk.

Chris wore a football helmet whenever he was on his crutches. One Sunday morning, after we had come home from church, we were all visiting on our front porch. Nobody was paying much attention to Chris, who was walking first here and then there—as a small child will do. Suddenly, he lost his balance and went backwards onto the tile porch floor, hitting his head with a terrible thud.

I grabbed him up in my arms—he was stunned. My heart was pounding in my chest; Mother ran for the phone. I'm sure that Uncle Charley broke every speed limit coming across town. He was on the porch, examining Chris, almost before Mother got back from the phone. Chris was crying by this time and his eyes looked odd. Uncle Charley felt that he had had a concussion. We were instructed to watch him very carefully and to keep him awake until late evening. I was to call at once if he should become nauseated.

We were lucky; by evening, Chris seemed to be all right except for the big lump on the back of his head. That went away in a few days; however, it was years after that before Chris was allowed to be on crutches without his helmet . . . you always "lock that stable after the horse is stolen."

Harry and I worked with Chris on the swing-through gait . . . Harry showed him the motion. He swang when he was in the bars, but when I put him out on the walk and told him to swing-through on the crutches, Chris refused. I found that if I took hold of the band on the back of his brace, he would do what I wanted. At first, I sort of helped him by lifting and pushing him slightly so that he got the feel of what he was supposed to be doing. It worked. He began to swing-through, with me holding the back of his brace. Soon I was no longer holding him; my hand was merely touching him. Every time I took my hand away, he would stop dead still. This procedure went on for some time.

One day, I decided that I would try to trick him. I picked up a stick that had fallen from the tree in the yard. As he started out walking, I had my hand on his brace; then I replaced it with the stick. He went cheerfully down the walk with me gently touching his back with the end of the stick. All at once he looked back and realized what was happening . . . Was he ever mad! He was so mad that big tears formed in his eyes as he fussed at me. I shouldn't do that! I was supposed to be holding him!

After I got him calmed down, I was able to get him to see that he had been walking—swinging-through—all by himself. He didn't need me or anybody else to hold him. He turned and walked back toward the house with a big grin on his face. He was as happy as the rest of the family, who had been watching from the porch to see what was going to happen. I had told them of my plan to try the stick.

After that experience, he walked most of the time with the swing-through gait. He was smart enough to realize that it was much faster and took a lot less effort.

Chris and I often took a walk on the sidewalks in our

neighborhood when the weather was nice. One particular evening, we walked up the hill toward the school which Art and Bob attended; then we decided to go on down the other side of the hill and around several blocks, mostly just to see what was on the other side. Even though we didn't see anything especially exciting or unusual, we enjoyed our walk into new territory. We were both exhausted when we got home, so Chris went to bed before very long.

The next morning, when I was dressing Chris, I noticed an enlarged place on his upper thigh, but I didn't pay much attention to it. We were scheduled to see Uncle Charley in a week or so . . . if it was not better by that time, then he'd see what the trouble was. Most of the swelling had disappeared by the time we saw Uncle Charley. He wanted the leg to be X-rayed. The X-ray revealed a clean fracture of the right femur, just below the hip. The bone appeared to be healing satisfactorily. No great damage had been done, thank goodness. I wondered how stupid I could be! I should have called Uncle Charley the minute that I noticed something different about Chris's leg. I could think of nothing that could have caused the break except that we probably walked about a mile or more that evening. As a precaution, we didn't walk that far again for a long time.

Harry had begun to teach Chris to go up and down steps. He had a set of steps at the center, with risers just about four inches high with an adjustable rail. He suggested that we have something similar at home. Jimmy built a set of steps over the back porch steps. We had metal rails built for the back and front porch steps. The top rail was built to standard adult height. There was a lower rail added that could be raised one inch at a time. So began the development of a new skill.

It did not take Chris long to master the four-inch steps. He could then almost make it in and out of the house by himself. He couldn't manage the screen door, but how many three-year-olds can get in and out of a screen door by themselves?

Most of my friends were beginning to send their children

to nursery school. Dr. Williams and Uncle Charley both told me they felt that we should begin to try to find a school that would take him. Chris needed to be around children his own age.

So, I began making the rounds of schools that friends recommended. Each director was very nice, but each had some excuse. The school was full, the personnel could not handle a child who was not toilet trained, or they were afraid the other children might hurt him. Not one would say that the school would try him for even a few days.

Uncle Charley told me that the local college was planning a nursery school as a part of its new teacher-training school. He suggested that I apply there immediately, before the classes were filled. At the time, I was involved with the PTA at the state level. I knew the state vice-president was a department chairman at the college, the department of teacher training which would be in charge of the new school. We often traveled to meetings together, so I discussed with him the possibility of Chris's attending the new school. He did not see any problems and told me that he would put my name on the list to receive applications. He pointed out that applications would be accepted in the order in which they were received.

I returned the completed application form the same day that I received it in the mail. I was confident that Chris would be accepted for the school.

I began to hear from friends that so-and-so was going to campus school. Surely my letter of acceptance for Chris would come in a few days. After a week or two, I felt that something was wrong. I called my friend at the college and he said that he could not imagine what had happened, but that I should talk to the gentleman who had been hired as the principal of the school. I called. He did not recall seeing Chris's application, but if I had sent it in when I said I did, then the teacher probably had it and my letter of acceptance probably was lost. I should call the teacher. I called.

No, she did not have Chris's application. But I had mailed

it months ago! Couldn't she possibly take him? He would be just one more. Then began the excuses . . . a step between the rooms that the class would be using, the unpreparedness to handle children who were not toilet trained . . . On and on went the reasons why she could not accept Chris.

I was furious. What she was really telling me was that she was afraid to handle a child who did not appear to be physically like every other child. Here was a state supported school which was supposed to train teachers, and the school was afraid to handle a child who was different. How were new teachers ever going to learn to teach these children!! Fortunately, the philosophy of the school has since changed, and it now has a very outstanding program for training teachers of the handicapped.

Where did I go from here? If this were the attitude that I got at nursery school, what would happen when Chris was old enough to go to public school? So often, Harry and I had discussed the fact that Chris was a bright little guy and would have to compete in the world with those who did not have visible handicaps. The sooner he began this competition, the better he would be able to cope with it. He needed to attend public school.

At the time, both Uncle Charley and I were serving on the Harrisonburg Recreation Commission. The commission had hired a young, enthusiastic director, who had developed a rapidly growing program. He asked the commission to hire a female assistant to help him with the program for girls and adults. Shortly after the new assistant was hired, I suggested that the community needed a nursery school type of activity, for those children whose parents could not afford the price of the private nursery school. It would give young mothers a chance to get out of the house and to enjoy shopping or some program of planned recreation that the department might offer.

The new assistant thought that suggestion was a good idea, and she started working on the details. She agreed to take Chris into the program, which met three days a week.

It was just what the doctor ordered. Chris looked forward to the days at the recreation center. There were fifteen to twenty other children in the program, including Uncle Charley's daughter, who had originally been enrolled at the campus nursery school.

The children accepted Chris without any question. It was almost eight months before even one of them wanted to know why he was wearing braces. After a simple answer from the young recreation supervisor that he needed them to walk, they asked no more questions.

For almost two years, Chris attended the Tiny-Tots program at the recreation department. It was as good a program as any of the nursery schools offered in town at that time. The program met a need in the community, and it is still part of the offerings of the recreation department of the city.

I continued working with the parents' group at the center, as well as serving as a member of the board. The parents and the center staff felt that their handicapped children needed to associate with other children who were not members of their own families. Since most of these children were not able to attend public school, we discussed the question of how such associations might be arranged. It was decided that we would establish a day camp at a local resort that offered its facilities for several days during one week in the summer. The program was open to all of the families and any friends who wanted to attend. We were able to find people in the community who volunteered their time to come each morning and to work with the children, by teaching them various craft skills and helping with them in the swimming pool. The first year that we held this day camp, we were at a resort having no luncheon facilities, so each family brought a picnic lunch. The next year, another resort offered its facilities, and it furnished meals. After that, for two summers, we turned the day camp into a family camping weekend. The resort made cabins available and furnished meals. It was great for all of the children, the handicapped and the nonhandicapped. It was great, too, for the parents, for many of them had not been able to have any type of vacation since the birth of their handicapped child, as they had no one to care for the child. Everyone came to the realization that their family was not the only family which had a different child with special problems. The sharing, loving, and understanding shown during those weekend camping sessions were great. Many friendships were formed that have lasted many years.

For several years, Harry helped us set up and carry out these camping sessions, but he left the center to enter medical school. Even though he had four children by this time, and was in his midthirties, he succeeded in gaining admission to medical school and finally realized a longtime dream. He had married early and had settled for a career in physical therapy, but he had not lost that burning desire to be a doctor.

Shirley, a new physical therapist, took his place. Shirley came to the center shortly after Harry had left. She was able to continue with the program that he had established. Shirley was married to a young man hired to work as the physical therapist at the local hospital. Often, they took Chris or other children from the center on outings. They took Chris to the golf course with them. Chris thought that this sport was great. They rented a golf cart and let Chris ride around the course with them.

Since several of the children at the center had had polio, I also got involved in working for the March of Dimes. I had also been involved in that work through the Parent Teachers' Association. One year, I was asked to be the fund drive chairman, and I accepted. That year, the drive was quite successful; later I was asked to serve as the local chapter chairman. I accepted. In working with the local media and March of Dimes regional personnel, I revealed that I had a son with a birth defect. About this time, the National Foundation (March of Dimes) was beginning to work on the causes of birth defects, because the polio vaccine had been developed and it was doing a great job in wiping out polio. The National Foundation Public Relations Office contacted us to see if we would mind their using Chris for some public relations photos. I talked it over with Jimmy, and we decided that if other people could be helped by Chris, then we would cooperate in any way that we could.

So, a photographer and a writer came to Harrisonburg to follow Chris and me around for a week. When he heard the story of how we had all walked on crutches to get Chris to walk, he wanted a picture. Along with a story, the picture was used in newspapers all over the country. I received letters from parents of spina bifida children from many different parts of the country. I tried to write to each one, giving them some information or help in any way that I could.

I talked with Dr. Williams about the kind of things that I should tell these people who were hoping and searching for something for their child. He pointed out I should always make it very clear that every spina bifida is different. One child's involvement is never exactly the same as another's. Therefore, what works for one will not always work for another. The parent should find a doctor in whom they have faith and confidence, and follow his instructions as best they possibly can.

The writer almost ate and slept with us. He took pictures everywhere we went and of everything we did. He decided that Chris might be a good candidate for the national poster child. The idea was kind of exciting, so we agreed that he might be considered. One of the pictures was taken in a wheelchair, which was borrowed, because Dr. Williams had said, "No wheelchair."

A pretty little girl was selected to be the national poster child that year. We were told that Chris was runner-up. A minute girl, with braces below her frilly dress, was thought to have more appeal than a little boy in short pants with his braces showing.

I'm sure that one of the reasons Chris was selected as a candidate was the fact that he bubbled with personality. He always had a smile, and I don't think he has ever seen a stranger. He will strike up a pleasant conversation with anyone he meets.

I shall never forget, one day, when we were in a department store in Richmond, after one of the frequent visits to see Dr. Williams. Usually, Chris and I stopped in one of the stores to get lunch. Chris was no different from most small children, and he wanted me to buy him every toy that he saw. This, of course, was impossible. I usually gave him a small amount of money and let him shop around until he found something that he wanted to buy. This time, it was a dollar more than he could afford. He asked for more money and I refused, because this situation had happened before. He needed to learn that he could not always have just what he wanted. Again, as many children do, he began to fuss and the fussing turned to tears. I continued to say "no" and I walked away from him. That was when the "dear little old lady" walked up to him and gave him a dollar. I was disgusted. . . . I chalked that one up to experience and Chris got the toy that he wanted.

After we got out of the store, I told him that if he cried or made a fuss about not having enough money the next time we went to the store, that would be the last time I would take him shopping for a long time. Next trip he was very cooperative.

Chris often went to the grocery store with me, walking on his crutches. At times, when he put his crutches in the basket and walked by holding onto the basket, he told me that he was helping me to push the basket. I had to be careful to keep a hand on the basket, so that it did not get away from him. Sometimes, when he was on his crutches, he would fall. I let him get up by himself. If I did not happen to be close by, well-meaning peole would rush to pick him up. I'm sure that, many times, people thought that I was very heartless. Chris had been taught to fall and to get up. He knew exactly how to do it. When someone took hold of him, it was done in such a way that Chris could not use his arms. People did not realize that he had to use his arms as legs. When he couldn't use his arms, he couldn't stand.

One of the funniest falls that Chris ever took was on the

sidewalk, in front of the house. One summer afternoon, shortly after a hard thundershower, the Good Humor man came around the corner with his bell ringing, signaling to all of the neighborhood children. Chris wanted a chocolate cone. His Daddy has always had a hard time telling Chris, or any of the boys, he could not have something. So, he went across the street to get the cone for Chris. Chris waited patiently on the corner until his Dad returned. Then Dad suggested that Chris should go and sit on the porch to eat the cone. There was a large puddle of mud on the walk between the corner and the house. Chris was flying, for he was in a hurry to consume the ice cream before it melted.

His crutches hit the mud; he went down, face first into the mud. Such a mess I have never seen. Jimmy yelled for me to get the ice cream and put it in the freezer. He picked Chris up and put him, braces, crutches, and all, into the tub. As soon as most of the mud was cleared away from his face and hands, he got to sit in the tub and eat the cone. He was happy as he could be. All of the mud did not bother him.

Chris and I had good times shopping together and doing errands together. One day, it was necessary for me to take my car into the garage for servicing. There was a waiting room for the customers, and I sat down to read. Chris didn't want to sit down; he wanted to go into the office and talk to the manager who was a friend of our family. Somehow or other he succeeded in convincing the manager to take him out into the shop, where they were working on our car. Chris always wanted to be where the action was. Well, this time there was a lot of action! He accidently placed one of his crutches on a greasy spot on the floor. . . . Down he went into a big tray of crankcase oil that had just been drained from my car. Man, was he ever a mess! Black oil from head to foot. I had on a beautiful, handknit sweater that he immediately grabbed with his black, greasy, little hand. The garage men covered the seat and floor of my car with plastic, and helped me to get him into the car. Once again, he went into the tub, braces and all.

Another day, we were going to the grocery store and we noticed that there was a train car off of the track. Naturally, Chris wanted to see what was happening. I didn't object a lot, because I like the action, too. We pulled off of the street, just across from where the train car was located. We sat there for some time, watching the men go about the job of getting it back on the track.

When the work no longer seemed to be so interesting, I started the car motor and pulled, at least I started to pull, into the line of traffic. From out of nowhere came a car that collided with the front fender of my car. Fortunately, no one was injured and my car was only slightly damaged. The other car received considerable damage. The police and insurance man were called. I stayed in the car with Chris until the policeman came to the side of the car to talk with me.

Chris greeted the officer with, "It's all Judy's fault!" For once, I almost wished that he could not verbalize so well. Thank goodness the policeman did not realize I was the Judy that Chris was referring to, because my legal name of Julia appeared on my driver's license.

I do not recall a single time when we had an appointment with Dr. Williams that we have not made the trip down to Richmond. We always kept the appointment—whether the weather was rain, shine, snow, or sleet. One winter day, we got up very early to make the trip to Richmond, for the weather report had called for snow and freezing rain. It was one of those times when the weather man happened to be correct. It took us at least an hour longer than usual. When we arrived in Richmond, we placed Chris in his stroller, which we used occasionally in places where we needed to move through traffic or when we needed to get someplace in a hurry. It was a struggle getting from the parking lot across the street to Dr. Williams's office at MCV, but we made it through the ice and snow.

We were dumbfounded when we walked into the office area and found it deserted. There was no one anywhere. I was sure that I had the right day, but I checked the appointment card in my bag. We had the correct day. I went into the office next door to see if the staff knew anything about Dr. Williams.

There, I found out we were supposed to have been notified that Dr. Williams was out of the office for several days, attending a conference on bracing. His secretary, who was not very efficient, was taking the days off, but she had failed to notify us. She was a lovely person, but she felt her main responsibility was to entertain the patients. The gentleman whom I talked to could see that I was upset, as I explained to him our driving through really rough weather conditions to keep the appointment.

He offered to phone Dr. Williams, to find out if there was any possibility that he could see Chris. Fortunately, the conference was being held, there, at the Medical College of Virginia. When the gentleman returned from talking to Dr. Williams, we were instructed to follow him. We were led into the elevator, to an underground tunnel that connected all of the buildings which were part of the Medical College of Virginia. We walked for quite a distance before we entered another elevator and went up several floors. There, we were led into a large room and told that Dr. Williams would meet us there in a few minutes.

He appeared from an adjoining room, and asked that I bring Chris into the room. As I entered, I saw the longest table that I think I have ever seen. Around the table were men seated at microphones. Many people were standing around the edge of the room. Some had on the white coats that doctors wear in the hospital. I recognized two of the men seated near the room's entrance, for I had seen their pictures in Easter Seal and National Foundation publications. One was Dr. Deavers, the New York doctor, and the other Dr. Bennett, the head of the Warm Springs, Georgia Foundation. Dr. Williams put Chris up on the table with his crutches and asked that he take a few steps. He did, and Dr. Williams explained the bracing, and reported a brief medical history of Chris to those present. Several of the others that were sitting around the table got up and came to examine Chris.

I shall never forget Dr. Deavers saying, "What in the hell do you have those crutches on him for?" It was true the he needed new crutches, having outgrown the pair that he was using. This replacement was to have been one of the things to be done on that trip to Richmond. Dr. Deaver's remark sparked a heated discussion among several of the men, including Dr. Williams. Through this experience, I realized that doctors often have differences of opinion about how to treat the patient. In many cases, they are working on past successes or trying out what seems to be a logical treatment process.

We learned later, that the men attending this bracing conference were the top men in the field, from the most outstanding medical schools in the eastern part of the United States. We had secured medical advice that probably could not have been brought together if we had had a countless amount of money. I still feel that God must have been working for us. How else would both Dr. Williams and the secretary forget to notify us about his being out of the office? All of his other patients had been notified.

Many times during the years, when Dr. Williams has watched Chris as he walks, he has remarked, "Damn it! Those crutches work!" Yes, they surely do!

Around the time that Chris was three years old, Dr. Williams felt that another doctor should be added to the team of specialists who were working with Chris. Dr. Williams explained that there were many urologists in Richmond, but he felt Chris should be under the care of someone who understood the special problems of the paraplegic. He recommended Dr. Henry Samuels of Staunton, because he had treated patients at Woodrow Wilson Rehabilitation Center with considerable success. Dr. Williams and Dr. Samuels were concerned that the weakness in Chris's bladder could cause serious infections and eventually kidney damage, if something were not done.

Dr. Samuels was able to keep infections to a minimum

through the use of mycine drugs. At that time, they were very expensive. The druggist was most helpful and suggested that if we bought them in hundred-lot bottles, he could give us a sizeable discount. The hundred lot was only a month's supply. Chris was good about taking capsules, but we found that he needed to take a glass of milk before he took the capsule or he would get a stomach pain.

Dr. Samuels ordered an annual IV polygram to keep check on how Chris's bladder was functioning. He explained that the bladder was weak, and it sometimes failed to empty properly. There was a possibility of the urine backing up into the kidneys. He felt that surgery would be necessary, sometime before Chris was much older. It occurred to me that maybe the surgery would have to be done in the summer, or Chris would have to miss school. If all went well, he would start school in the fall.

VII

Chris was five years old and ready to begin attending public school almost before I could realize it. As his brothers before him, he had a birthday party the year he was five. He invited all of his friends from Tiny-Tots. They had a great time playing games and eating ice cream and cake.

The local superintendent of schools was a member of the Crippled Children's Rehabilitation Center board, the new name given to the Cerebral Palsy Clinic where Chris had received physical therapy treatments. I knew that he understood the problems of educating those children who were different. I discussed Chris's educational plans with him at length. We both felt that Chris should attend the public schools. He said Chris could be enrolled in any of the schools in the city that I wanted to select. One school that was all on one floor was recommended as probably best for Chris. Jimmy and I talked it over. We decided that Chris should attend the neighborhood school his brothers had attended. True, it meant that he would have steps and a lot of them, but we felt this mastering of steps was part of his learning experience. The world would not stop building buildings with steps just because Chris Grandle could not go up the steps. Chris's bedroom was located on the second floor of our house, even though there is a room on the first floor which could have been converted into a bedroom for him. He had learned to walk up the standard size step, and the little steps that Jimmy had built at the back door of the house had been taken down.

Chris and I have often remarked that he was so fortunate

Harry taught him to go up steps backward. Many physical therapists teach their patients to go up the steps forward. This approach does not give them the security that they need on steps, making the learning process much harder, especially for young children. It is also much more dangerous to walk up the steps forward on crutches, because there is no way to catch yourself if you should start to fall. When backing up the steps, if you start to fall, you simply sit down on the steps.

During Chris's first year in public kindergarten, the class was held in a room on the ground floor. He had no problems at all. The class met only for two and a half hours. He still wore his football helmet. All of the children in the class wanted their mothers to buy them football helmets. Even the little girls wanted to wear football helmets. The children in his class accepted Chris just the same way that the children of the Tiny-Tots had accepted him. They did not notice that he was different, only that he had a football helmet and they wanted one too.

Chris was beginning to have problems with his tonsils, as many children of five do. Dr. Samuels also said he felt that it was time for surgery to construct the reimplantation of the urethra. This operation could prevent the urine from backing up into the kidneys from the bladder. We felt Chris's hospitalization should be in the spring, after the close of school. He would be fully recuperated by the time school opened again in the fall. This would mean that we could not have our vacation with our friends at the beach as we had for the last several years.

Dr. Samuels agreed that I should go to the hospital to stay with Chris. I knew how to handle him and could care for him more easily than a special nurse could. I might also aid the floor nurses in caring for him.

On the pediatrics floor of the Staunton hospital at that time, no facilities existed for parents to stay with their children. Dr. Samuels arranged for a cot to be put in the room beside Chris's bed—one of those with a metal rail along each side, with flat springs, and covered with a thin mattress. When I lay on the cot, I sank down in the middle and had to climb over the rail to get out. Needless to say, it was not the most comfortable bed I'd ever slept in.

The doctors gave Chris the works on that trip to the hospital. He had his tonsils removed, he had the reimplantation, and he was circumcised. The doctor had failed to do the customary circumcision when he was born because he said that Chris would not live long anyway. Even with so much surgery, he got along fine. I found it was much easier to care for him now than it had been during those hospital days in Richmond. Jimmy came to see us each night, and Mom and the boys came sometimes during the day.

Chris recuperated rapidly and was ready to begin school in the fall. That year, his classroom was on the first floor of the building. He had to go up a flight of eight steps to get to that level of the building. Then, a short flight of three steps lead to another level, where the restrooms, clinic, and the principal's office were located.

Students in the first grade were required to stay until two o'clock. The children were allowed to come home for lunch or they could eat in the cafeteria, located on the ground floor.

Late in the summer, I went to school to discuss the problems involving Chris's attendance with the principal. He told me that Chris was to be placed with a teacher of much experience who had raised a large family of children. He felt that she would treat Chris like any other child and would not be afraid to cope with his handicap. I assured him that Chris could manage all of the steps involved, but that I thought it might be well for him to be allowed to go up or down the steps when there was not so much traffic on the steps. The principal agreed.

The only thing that I could see would cause a problem, was that Chris could not control his bladder or his bowels. I suggested that this problem be solved by my coming to school each day at midmorning and just before lunch, to take care of his toilet needs. As a result of my suggestion, the principal arranged that Chris and I would use the private restroom in the clinic, just off of the principal's office. Disposable pads were now available for the plastic panty he wore. I had learned to change the pads quickly and efficiently when Chris was standing up. I no longer needed to go through the long process of removing his braces.

Everything seemed to be working out fine during the first few days of school. Then, one morning Chris said that he was sick. His stomach hurt. He didn't want to go to school. I kept him home that day, but I noticed that it was not long before he seemed to feel great. I didn't think much about it that day.

The next morning Chris was sick again—all the same symptoms. When he got to feeling better about midmorning, I decided to take him to school. He got along fine.

The same thing was repeated for two more mornings. Finally, I decided to take him to the emergency room at the hospital for Uncle Charley to check him over. He could see if anything were wrong with Chris . . . or if something at school were bothering him.

Uncle Charley declared that Chris was "fit as a fiddle," and that there was absolutely no reason for him having a "pain" in his stomach. Consequently, Jimmy and I began to ask questions, trying to discover from Chris if something was wrong that he didn't want to go to school in the morning, but was perfectly willing to go later in the day.

Our questioning led to a discovery. A classmate had told Chris that the principal of the school could burn up the school and all the children when he wanted to, and that he would blow the fire alarm before he did. This particular classmate, who was repeating first grade, had a great need to be recognized and accepted. She found that by telling the younger children wild tales they would look up to her and think she was great.

We told Chris there was no truth in what this child was telling him, but, nevertheless, she had instilled a real sense of fear in Chris. His teacher assured him that she would never allow him to be left in the building. She would just grab him up like a sack of flour—she did, too, whenever they had a fire drill. She lived on a farm and was used to handling sacks of feed. Even this procedure did not settle his fear. We discovered he was smart enough to analyze the procedure for fire drills at the school. It provided that the drills be held every day during the first two weeks of school each year, and that they be held during the first hour or so of the day. This fact explained why he felt sick in the morning and was then willing to go about midmorning; the fire drills would be over.

To assist Chris's independence, Jimmy hit on the idea that if there were a rail for Chris to use at the steps leading out the front of the building, Chris could then get out himself. We asked permission of the school to place rails on either side of those steps. They agreed, as long as we paid for the materials and furnished the labor. Jimmy did a professional job of installing the rails . . . another problem solved. Chris no longer felt he was trapped in that building. In later years, and in classes that met on the second floor of the building, a team of four large boys would be assigned to carry him out of the building when a fire drill occurred. They would practice periodically when no one was using the steps. As a result, both the boys and Chris felt comfortable and confident when the fire drills were held.

Dr. Samuels continued to treat Chris with medication to keep down infection. He felt that another reimplantation was needed in the other urethra. This time there was no cot. In its place I found a recliner. I didn't know how I would get along with that for a bed. The nurse gave me a pillow for my head and a light blanket to cover up. I learned that if I put the pillow under my bottom instead of my head, I was in a prone position and could sleep with little discomfort. In fact, I came to the conclusion that the recliner was more comfortable than the cot. The hospital staff admitted that the cots had finally all collapsed and been thrown out.

Chris had a total of three reimplantations during his elementary years. In the third operation, both urethras were reimplanted. Dr. Samuels said he wanted to try one more time to get a successful reimplantation. He explained that another operation could be performed, but it was irreversible. He was afraid that "it would burn our bridges behind us." He felt perhaps we could buy some time, during which new surgical techniques might be developed that would not "burn the bridges."

During these stays in the hospital, Chris learned to know a lot of the patients and the hospital staff. They all loved him and stopped by to see him frequently. As soon as he could be up in a chair, he wanted to go up and down the hall to visit those who could not get out of their rooms.

In the meantime, Dr. Samuels said he thought that Chris was large enough to be fitted with a urinal. We tried some of the commercial products that the doctor recommended. Chris was just too little, or the urinals were too big. They slipped off or they leaked. We tried everything we could think of. One day, I even tried the substance that is sold to keep false teeth in place, thinking that it might work for Chris—no luck! We really had a time. Dr. Samuels suggested that I improvise by purchasing prophylactics, then taping one securely to a tube that ran into a small bag strapped around his leg. I made small elastic rings to slip up over his penis to hold the top of the prophylactic in place. The elastic ring was about as big around as my second finger. Problem—how can I get that ring into place? More tears from Chris . . . I cried too. It was very frustrating for both Chris and me as I tried to get that equipment into place. Dr. Samuels didn't have any further suggestions.

Dear Jimmy came up with the answer. On the farm, a four-pronged instrument was used to slip a rubber band in place when lambs were castrated. He brought this home for us to try. It worked slick as a whistle. Chris no longer needed to wear the plastic panty with the diaper insert. He had almost grown too large for those available on the market. He also had established a time schedule for his bowel movements. Once in a while he had an accident and needed to change.

Sometimes, the urinal would slip out of place, then he had to have help, but by the time that Chris was in fourth grade he was able to take care of his own toilet needs. I no longer needed to make the trips to school to take him to the rest room.

The urinal and the lift on his right shoe caused us to make some modifications in Chris's clothing. Because of his brace, his pant legs could not be rolled high enough to empty the bag that was strapped on his leg. With the help of a local seamstress, zippers were put into each leg of his pants, solving the problems that we encountered.

For years, I carried a pair of the four-pronged openers in my handbag. Dr. Samuels said he hoped no one needed to search my handbag. I would certainly cause some questions! I seriously doubt that many people would recognize the instrument that I carried.

Chris outgrew the stroller we had used for many years to take him where he could not walk, because of crowds or distance. Dr. Williams finally consented for us to buy a wheelchair for Chris. We also purchased a small roll-about chair for use in the house. He used that instead of sliding around on the floor. It did save a lot of washing. Dr. Williams cautioned that we were not to let him use either chair as a substitute for his walking.

The summer of the New York World's Fair, we decided to take Chris and Bob to New York. Art had been able to find a summer job in a local factory that summer, and he could not get off. I told Dr. Williams of our plans to attend the fair. He had been there the month before, and he insisted that we take Chris's wheelchair. I could not understand this instruction; he never wanted Chris to use a chair. I complained that we planned to use commercial transportation from the hotel to the fairgrounds. I didn't see how we could manage a chair. Then Dr. Williams explained that there were rental chairs available at the fair.

I was still very puzzled by this sudden turn in Dr. Williams.

We arrived at the gate of the fair which Dr. Williams had

instructed us to use, and found the place to rent Chris a chair. Then, we started out to see the fair. The lines were just as long as we had heard they would be, but we decided that we might as well join one if we were going to see anything.

We had stood in line only a few minutes when a young uniformed attendant came up to us. He wanted to know how many were in the party. We told him that there were four of us. He instructed us to bring Chris and follow him. We went around to the side of the exhibit building; there, he unlocked a door and took us in. Within a few minutes, we were viewing the exhibit we had expected to wait at least an hour to see.

Gee! That was great. . . . We were sold on the product responsible for that exhibit. They were so nice to us with the VIP treatment.

We picked another exhibit and took our place in the line in front of the exhibit. Once again, we were met after just a few minutes by a young, uniformed attendant. Again we were taken in a side entrance and given the VIP treatment. Suddenly, I understood what Dr. Williams had been trying to tell us. We found the wheelchair to be the magic key. Each time that we stood in a line to enter an exhibit, we were greeted by a young attendant and taken in a side or rear entrance. We saw far more at the fair then the average person who was there only three days.

Several other interesting things happened while we were in New York. We had told our friend, the writer with the National Foundation, that we would be in New York to see the fair. The New York Yankees were playing at home during this time. The National Foundation arranged for us to have box seats at a game in the old Yankee Stadium. They wanted to arrange for Chris to have his picture taken before the game with Mickey Mantle. This picture could not be arranged, because it took several hours for the trainer to tape Mickey Mantle's legs before the game. However, Chris went down onto the field before the game with the National Foundation representatives and met several of the players. Tony Kubek posed with him for a picture, which appeared in the New York papers the next day. It was put on the wire service and used across the nation. The local paper also ran the picture. Chris was more concerned about getting the autographed baseball that the team promised than seeing his picture in the paper.

The next day we decided to take a tour of the United Nations before leaving New York. As we walked through the large lobby of the United Nations, I was behind Chris. I happened to notice, that as he walked, two small, marblelike objects fell from his pants leg. I recognized the familiar little balls, quickly stooped, picked them up with a tissue, and headed for the nearest trashcan. I'm sure that only the family knew what had happened. We all had to laugh, because Chris is probably the only person in the world who had done such a thing on the floor of the United Nations building and gotten away with it.

On the way home from New York, we stopped for several days at the beach. In the motel room next to ours, we discovered a high school classmate of Jimmy's whom he had not seen since their graduation. Tom was vacationing with his family for a week. He was then working in Baltimore, and his next-door neighbor was Brooks Robinson. Chris, thrilled by the fact that he could actually talk to someone who actually knew Brooks Robinson, told them about his visit to Yankee Stadium and about the autographed ball that they had promised to send him. He was wondering if Tom could get Brooks Robinson to send him an autographed ball from the Baltimore Orioles. Tom promised he would try. Sure enough, one day, shortly after we got home from vacation, a package, along with a letter from Brooks Robinson, arrived for Chris. It was the baseball Tom had promised!

Chris tried to do anything that Bob or Art could do. There were many things they could do, but they were not always so willing to do them, such as mowing the lawn. Art always argued about doing it when he was asked to help out. Bob just seemed to not hear and got lost very quickly. But Chris decided that he would like to mow the lawn, especially after Jimmy bought a riding mower.

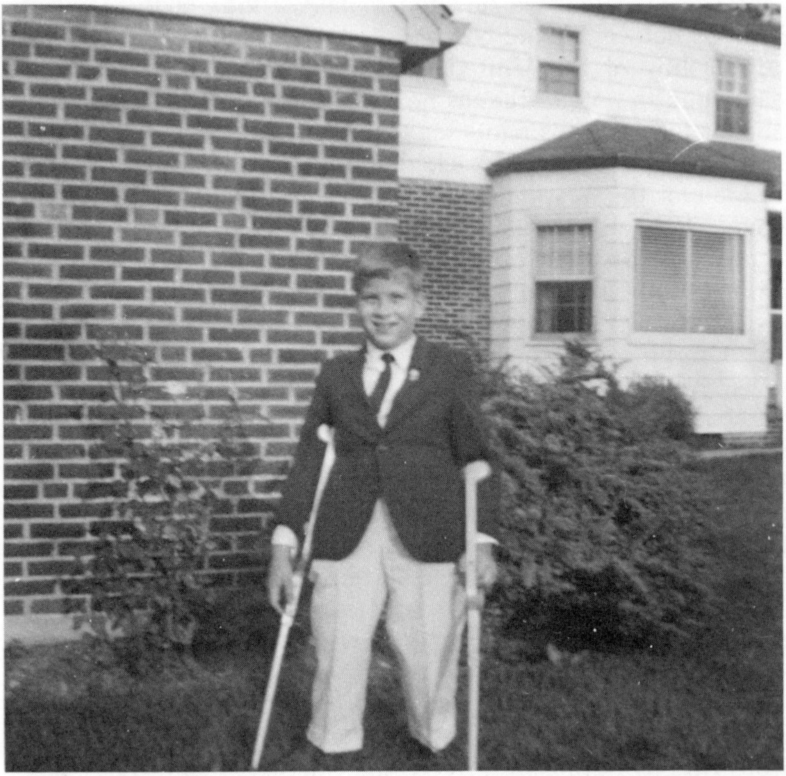

The Easter Sunday that Chris joined the church (he was nine years old).

We rarely ever told Chris that he could not try to do something, so Jimmy helped him get on the mower and showed him how he should drive around the edge of the lawn, getting closer to the center on each round. Those directions were much too orderly for Chris. He felt that a better way to mow the lawn would be to just go round in circles in a haphazard fashion. Jimmy tried to show him the way that he thought it should be done. Chris could not see any fun in doing the lawn that way; however, he did decide finally that he would do it as Daddy wanted it done. Unfortunately, after helping with the lawn once or twice during the hot summer days, Chris followed Bob's example. When the lawn needed mowing, Chris got lost! No more was ever said about wanting to ride Daddy's power mower.

In the fall of 1963, Art went to college. I had made both of the older boys a bargain some years before, that if they would help me to get my master's degree by taking care of Chris and the house while I was at school, that I would see that they got to go to college. I had been doing substitute teaching ever since Bob and Art started to school. I had not thought that I wanted to be a teacher when I was an undergraduate student, but I started substituting because my own children were in classes which did not always have a teacher. I liked it. Then I worked with the PTA, trying to do something about the many unqualified teachers who were in the classrooms at that time. If I were going to teach, I had to go to school to earn my certification. Art and I both graduated the same June. He got his high school diploma, and I got my master's degree.

I started teaching at the local high school the fall that Art entered the School of Engineering and Applied Science of the University of Virginia. The principal was most understanding and assured me that if Chris should need me at any time, I could be released to go and take care of his needs. There were only a few times when he called me. Bob picked him up after school and took him home. During the days when I had substituted, Mom filled in for me by going to school and taking care of him.

On a lovely, fall, Sunday afternoon, when Chris was in the sixth grade, we took the family and drove to Blackwater Falls. The colors in the mountains that we crossed were beautiful. The leaves were orange, red, and gold, mixed with the dark green of the pine and spruce. We found that it was necessary to walk down several hundred steps in order to view the falls. Jimmy and the boys wanted to take the walk, but I thought I would remain at the top of the steps where Chris and I could sit enjoying the lovely colors. Chris would have no part of my plan. He was going with the boys to see the waterfall. He walked all of the way down and back up those steps, almost four hundred. He didn't seem to be even exhausted as we returned home late that evening.

It was in the middle of the night that I heard Chris screaming as though he were in severe pain. I went to see about him. He had pain in his back; he felt as though he had to go to the bathroom. He jumped out of his bed onto the floor to slide himself into the toilet. I heard a sound like a firecracker or a gun being fired, just as he hit the floor. As I looked at his leg lying out to the side of him in an odd position, I realized what the noise had been. Chris had broken his leg. I yelled frantically for Jimmy as I grabbed Chris's braces. As quickly and carefully as we could, we got him into his braces, to the toilet, and back to bed. He was having a lot of pain most of the night.

At the very crack of dawn, I spoke to Uncle Charley on the phone. He said that he didn't have any idea what to do about Chris's leg. He was afraid that the back pain was coming from a kidney infection. He prescribed a sedative and medication for the infection; then he suggested we call Dr. Williams and take Chris to Richmond.

Jimmy was able to obtain a stretcher from the local rescue squad for us to put Chris on, so that he could ride in the back of our station wagon. We stopped by the hospital pharmaceutical department and picked up the medication, before we started out for Richmond on a damp, drizzling, gloomy day.

Dr. Williams, now in private practice in the west end of

Richmond, was in his office, and he saw Chris immediately. Jimmy and I carried him in on the stretcher, because each doctor had cautioned that Chris should not move any more than necessary. Dr. Williams felt he should be X-rayed, but we had to go to another doctor down the street. So, Jimmy and I took Chris on the stretcher to the radiologist down the street. There, we waited until he had completed the films and had talked to Dr. Williams. They decided that Chris should be seen by an orthopedic surgeon whose office was in midtown Richmond.

Off we went in the drizzling rain. Chris, still on the stretcher, went back into the station wagon. Soon, we arrived in midtown and tried unsuccessfully to find a parking place. Finally, we stopped in the street long enough to get Chris out of the car, into the elevator, and up to the doctor's fifth-floor office, where Chris and I waited until Jimmy went back down to move the car out of the middle of traffic on the city street.

We waited a considerable amount of time. The receptionist had told us that the doctor was at the hospital, but she was expecting him at any time. Finally, she came out and said that the doctor wanted us to come down to the emergency room at the Medical College of Virginia.

So, we reversed our steps, carrying Chris, still on the stretcher and being extremely patient, back into the car and to the emergency room at MCV. There, he was examined by a resident who said that he would get in touch with the surgeon. We waited again. It was getting near midafternoon, when a nurse finally told us that the surgeon, Dr. Hammer, would see us back at his office just as soon as we could get there. Needless to say, Jimmy and I were about worn out, both physically and mentally. Chris was doing fairly well. The sedative had relieved his back pain, and he had no sensation in his leg.

About four o'clock that afternoon, Dr. Hammer finally saw Chris, went over the X-rays, and examined the area of his back where he had pain. His leg was definitely broken. All of the doctors seemed to agree on that point. It was a long spiral break of the right femur, about midway between his knee and his hip. Dr. Hammer said he felt that there was little that could be done, except to keep him in his braces for six weeks. They were not to be taken off for any reason. Chris was to use a chair and stay off his leg. In the meantime, we should see Dr. Samuels as soon as possible. Dr. Hammer explained that he could put Chris's leg in a cast, but we had done exactly the right thing when we put him in his braces after the accident. Jimmy and I had set the leg as well as any of the doctors. There was much less chance of Chris's developing pressure sores if his brace were used to hold the leg in place than if a cast were used. Using the braces would also be much easier for me to handle Chris. I could get a hold on the braces to lift him, whereas it was much more difficult to get hold of a cast.

Jimmy found that he could put a padded board on the roll-about chair we had at the house for Chris. This pad would serve as a leg rest, and the chair could be taken with him to school. It would also be easy for several large boys to carry him up and down the stairs to class. So, Chris was back in school the next day.

Dr. Samuel saw him several days later; he told me that the time had come when Chris needed more extensive surgery. He was not prepared or equipped to do it, so he wanted us to see a doctor at the University of Virginia who specialized in children's urinary problems.

Chris was admitted to the University of Virginia Hospital in November, just about five weeks after he had broken his leg. Dr. Hammer agreed that the brace could be removed long enough for surgery, provided an orthopedic specialist at the University supervised the handling of his leg while it was out of the brace.

After several days of tests, the doctor called me into his office to explain the proposed surgical procedure. The urethra implantations had not been successful in preventing the backward flow of urine into the kidneys. At that time, no permanent damage to the kidneys existed, but if the condition continued, irreparable and probably fatal damage would occur. The surgery proposed would cut off the bladder completely. A piece of the intestines would be used to make an opening to the outside wall of the abdomen. The urethra would be connected into this opening. The body waste collected by the kidneys would then empty through this opening in the abdomen wall. Chris would be properly fitted with a rubber appliance on his abdomen as soon as the surgery was properly healed. He estimated that Chris would be hospitalized about three weeks. One of my concerns was whether this operation would affect the reproductive system in any way. The doctor assured me it would not. Dr. Samuel had hinted that this was the operation that "burns the bridges." I had to ask what if . . . what if this doesn't work? At that time, there was nothing else that could be done. The doctor assured me that it had been successful in 90 percent or better of the cases. There was nothing else to do.

Chris and I were given a double room. I really had it made, in comparison to the other times when we had been hospitalized. It was decided that I would stay with Chris for the first few days after surgery, until I knew the worst was over. Then, Mom would drive to Charlottesville in the morning, while I drove to my teaching job in Harrisonburg. She stayed with Chris during the day; I left just as soon as my classes were through and went back to stay with him during the rest of the afternoon and until the next morning. I commuted between Charlottesville and Harrisonburg for almost two weeks.

Bob and Art were both in school in Charlottesville. They dropped by every evening to see us. Many times, they brought a group of friends with them. Chris thought this attention was great. One day, the orthopedist arranged for about five of the members of the University of Virginia football team to come to see him. He was quite a fan of the University of Virginia team; often, we had arranged to attend the football games in Scott Stadium while the boys were in college.

During his stay in the hospital, disposable plastic bags

were used over the stoma—the opening that had been made in his abdomen wall. To get these bags applied so that they would not leak was quite difficult. I seemed to be able to do it more efficiently than most of the nurses who were assigned to that floor. They said I was a much better "plumber" than they were. It got to the point that they tried to avoid changing the plastic bag until I arrived from school each afternoon. Actually, I discovered that the secret was making sure that Chris's skin was absolutely dry in the area where the adhesive on the plastic bag was to be applied.

Before Chris was released in time to be home for the Thanksgiving holidays, the resident measured his stoma and fitted him with a permanent appliance. I was given instructions on how to apply it. In the beginning, it was to be changed every day—then, every other day, then every third day; and so one, until he got to the point where he could wear it a week at a time. I was cautioned that the gradual build-up was to help prevent skin irritations from developing, because many people have sensitive skin, and the adhesive causes a rash or even rawness in that area.

At first, I began to wonder how we would find the time to take proper care of this equipment. It took me about forty-five minutes to change the appliance, but somehow we managed. The doctor gave us what was called a hospital kit of accessories for Chris's permanent appliance—it included a small sample bottle of glue and an equally small bottle of glue remover. The second time that I tried to change the appliance was on a holiday; I suddenly realized that the bottle of glue remover was almost empty. I sent Jimmy to the one drugstore that had remained open, for I was certain that you could just walk into any drugstore and purchase the necessary supplies. No one even knew what Jimmy was talking about, but after he described the situation to the druggist, the druggist suggested turpentine. It was not a very good substitute, but we made it do for that night. The next morning, Jimmy made a trip to Charlottesville to get a larger bottle of the glue and glue remover. For some years, we had to have our druggist order the supplies for us. As more and more people in the area had similar operations, the equipment became available to us.

Chris was delighted with his new appliance. He could now stand up to go to the bathroom, just like the other guys at school. He would no longer have to sit, empty the bag on his leg into a cup, and empty the cup into the toilet. He could use the "Boys" room at school and not have to use the restroom in the clinic as he had done before.

By the time he was discharged from the hospital for the surgery that constructed his ileal bladder, his leg was also healed enough that he could go back to school and resume his normal activity. Another benefit of the surgery was that he did not have to take any more medication for bladder infection.

Chris tried everything that everyone else did at school. One day, when he came home, I noticed that his right crutch was bent. I asked if he had fallen that day, for I thought maybe a crutch had gotten under him or hit something when he threw it out from under him. No, he hadn't fallen. What had he been doing that day?

He had been playing baseball. That was nothing new, for he had played many times before. "How did the crutch get bent?" I inquired rather impatiently.

He decided that the crutch would make a very good bat, then he could run the bases himself. He usually did the hitting, and then had someone else run the bases for him. If he had his crutch in his hand, he could start right on for first base. I suggested that he not do that anymore. The crutch was damaged enough that we had to buy a new pair.

The guys in his class at school were even willing for him to try playing football. He was not as successful at that sport—once or twice was enough. Both Bob and Art felt the same way about football.

Chris had learned to swim at the time when the parents held the day camp for children who attended the Rehabilitation Center. In the summer, we often visited friends who had a pool, so that Chris and I could swim. The pool had a plastic bottom, so at first, I did not dream that it would injure his feet. The first time he got out of the water, I noticed that he had rubbed the skin off the ends of all his toes. I had not been surprised when he had received a similar injury in a resort pool which had a concrete bottom. After this, I found that a pair of tennis shoes on his feet whenever he went swimming was the answer to keeping the skin on his toes. He had no feeling in his feet and never knew when he was hurt. When he was smaller, he had liked to hammer nails into a board as he had seen his Daddy and the boys do. We had to be very careful, for he could drive the nail through the board and into his leg without knowing he had done it.

One day, when we went to swim, our friend had the pool full of trout. He had bought them to put in a mountain pond under construction. The pond was not yet ready for fish, so he had the delivery truck put them in his swimming pool. Chris was given a fishing pole; he sat on the side of the pool and caught fish. He had a ball!

Some months later, when the pond was finished and the fish acclimated to their new surrondings, we went to see them. Our friend Bill told Chris that he could fish in the pond if he wanted to. Bill, his wife Mary, and I went off for a hike in the woods, leaving Jimmy and Chris on the bank of the pond fishing.

I was gripped with sudden terror as I heard Chris screaming. I ran through the woods toward the pond as fast as I could go, with Mary and Bill following me. I fully expected to see Chris in the water, or a big bear standing there, or something equally terrible. Instead, Chris was sitting there where we had left him, proudly holding up a large trout. It was much larger than the ones which had been put into the pond and was evidently a native trout. Both Chris and Jimmy were so excited that they almost jumped into the pond. Chris had been screaming because of his excitement. That was one fish which never reached the dinner table. We had to freeze it so that it could be taken to the taxidermist the next day. He mounted the fish, and we hung it proudly in the den.

VIII

Most summers, our family managed to find time for a vacation together. Chris was always included. We continued to go to the beach with our friends, until Chris was too heavy for us to carry across the sand to the ocean. The sun made the sand too hot for him to crawl, and sand ruined his braces. He was never satisfied to swim in a pool at the beach.. He had to be right out in the ocean with all of the other children. The summer that he was in the fourth grade, we went to Williamsburg as we had done with Bob and Art. We felt that the trip would make their study of Virginia's history much more interesting.

One summer, we went to Michigan with friends. Both families rented cottages on a lake where we could boat, fish, and swim. On the way to the lake, in the middle of the southern panhandle of Michigan, we decided to stop by the Ford Museum. As we entered, an attendant asked if we wanted a wheelchair for Chris, as there would be a lot of walking. One could see that Chris was too heavy to carry very far. I said I thought it might be a good idea. The attendant came with a very old-fashioned wheelchair, one of the high-backed, wooden kind that I remember seeing in the hospitals when I was a child. Chris had never seen anything like that, and he was not going to have any part of it. He would walk, and walk he did.

We had a great time seeing all of the old cars; then, we started into the exhibit of steam-powered vehicles, where some of the really big, old train engines were exhibited. All of a sudden, Chris stopped walking and said that he thought he had broken his brace; sure enough, it was broken! He had broken one of the upright pieces on the side.

Now, he would have to ride in that wheelchair. There were some tears, but I guess he saw that I was rather put out with him for not riding in the first place, so he cut them off short. I stayed with him until Jimmy went back to the entrance and requested a chair. The staff of the museum was so very helpful in aiding us in finding a brace repair shop that was not too far away. They called for us and made arrangements for Chris's brace to be repaired as soon as we could get to the shop. It took several hours for the repairs to be made, so we had to cut our tour of the museum short. Our friends were expecting us early that evening, and we had yet some distance to travel.

When I reflected on the experience, I guess that it was a good thing that the brace broke when it did. I'm sure that it would probably have broken sometime that week, and the lake was a long way from any place that we could have had the repairs made. God was looking after us, even if, at the time, I was a little doubtful about it.

Some years later, Jimmy, Chris, and I decided that we would tour the New England states. We enjoyed our trip very much—roaming through the New England countryside, stopping on the rugged coastline to look out over the Atlantic, and hunting out small restaurants that served unexcelled seafood. On the last day of the trip, we stopped to tour Sturbridge Village. At the gate, we were faced with a familiar scene.

The attendant asked Chris if he wanted a wheelchair. Remembering the time we had been in Michigan, both Jimmy and I insisted that Chris take the chair. Being the independent individual that he is, he was quite determined that he was going to walk.

We began the tour down the graveled pathways of the restored historical village. We had made it about halfway through the tour when Chris stopped. Both Jimmy and I had walked on ahead, and it was a minute or two before we were conscious of the fact that Chris was not with us. We both looked back about the same time and saw him standing in the middle of the path with a rather sheepish look on his face.

"Dad," he said, "would you mind going back to the gate and getting that wheelchair?"

"Why . . . what's wrong?" we both asked, almost at the same time.

"My brace is broken, and I'm afraid to walk any further on it."

We helped him to a nearby seat, where the two of us sat to wait until Jimmy went back to the main gate for a wheelchair. Unfortunately, that chair was not equipped with wide tires, so it was very difficult to push on the graveled paths. Even with Chris helping to move the chair, it was hard work for Jimmy and me to get him around. We cut the tour short, and began the final leg of the trip to visit Art, who was living in New Jersey.

There may have been a brace shop somewhere near Sturbridge Village, or in New York, but Jimmy and Art looked at the brace and decided they could make the repairs that were needed.

Many times during the years, Jimmy has made minor brace repairs or has repaired crutches so that Chris can function until an opportunity to take him to Richmond for the repairs occurred. Jimmy made the repairs without the benefit of the specialized equipment of the brace maker. I usually had to be his assistant and hold the braces while he made the repairs. Over the years, he has become very experienced in making these minor repairs.

The year that Chris was in the eighth grade, he experienced another broken leg. The year before, Dr. Williams felt that his back and hips had developed enough strength that the pelvic band could be removed from his braces. Chris had so much trouble with the brace breaking where it was attached to the band. He seemed to be able to maneuver quite well without the band. All appeared to be going well.

I had been elected as a delegate to the state education association meeting in Richmond. Mom said that she would look after Chris and the boys while I was gone. The second evening, as I was sitting in one of the meetings, listening not too intently to a speaker, my roommate slipped into the seat beside me and said that there was a man wanting to see me at the door. I was ever so surprised to see Dr. Williams. He informed me that he was going to take me to St. Mary's Hospital. Jimmy would be there with Chris until we got there.

What was wrong? What had happened?

Dr. Williams told me the story on the way through the city traffic. Chris had broken his leg at school. Jimmy had called, and Dr. Williams had told him to bring Chris to Richmond. Jimmy explained to the doctors where he could find me, so he came to get me while they were on the road.

Apparently, Chris had done something to his leg during the day, but he continued to walk on it until Mom picked him up at the close of school. He told her that he did not think his leg was just right; she called Jimmy, who was almost sure the leg was broken by looking at it. Chris had repeatedly said that the next time he went to the hospital, he wanted to go to St. Mary's. We always went past it as we traveled from the brace shop to Dr. Williams's West End Office. It was a beautiful, new, and appealing structure. Chris had told his Daddy to ask Dr. Williams if he could go there.

Dr. Williams ordered X rays taken, and then he called Dr. Hammer to come for a consultation. The femur was broken near the hip; again it was a straight, clean break that should not cause his leg to shorten as the earlier spiral break had done. The doctors decided again to let his brace serve as a cast. They saw no reason to admit him to the hospital.

We went by the hotel where I had been staying, picked up my things, and were home by midnight. Once again, the padded board was put on Chris's roll-about chair. I was able to find two high school boys willing to carry Chris up and down the steps at school. He did not miss one day of classes that time.

After his leg healed, the pelvic band was put back on his braces. Dr. Williams felt it was impossible for the leg brace to be tight enough to give the support near the tip of the femur bone. Chris's weight forced the hip backward, causing the bone to break.

Chris was hard on braces. At first, the braces were made of aluminum, but he managed to break them every few weeks. Jimmy made some of the repairs, but for others, we would have to make a trip to Richmond with Chris and his braces. The braces lasted only about eighteen months. They were designed to last at least three years. When the aluminum did not work, the brace makers tried steel. It was the same story. One pair he had exactly two weeks before he managed to break them. Each new pair was made from heavier and supposedly stronger material. Quarter-inch Chromolley steel was finally tried. When Chris went in to get that pair of braces, Tommy said, "We made two pair of these. One for Chris and one for the elephant in the circus." Naturally, he was being facetious, but the point he made was true. It seemed to me it would take an elephant to be able to carry those braces; they were so heavy. Tommy explained that the steel used in these braces was the same as that used in the construction of trucks. Surely, this metal would hold.

Tommy should have known Chris better than to think that. In three weeks, we were back in Richmond for repairs. Dr. Williams and Tommy just shook their heads. They didn't know what else to do. Chris didn't know what it meant to "take it easy." He went as hard and as fast as he could go.

Dr. Williams tried to persuade the National Institute of Health to accept Chris for testing new bracing materials with which they were experimenting. He felt that if a material would withstand Chris, it would take anything and anybody.

I could not help but think that there must be an answer somewhere. I just did not see how they could continue to make the braces heavier. I could barely lift them now with both hands. Chris didn't even seem to notice that he had them on.

It was about this time, in 1969, that Bob received his degree in aerospace engineering. It seemed that if he knew something about how to make an airplane fly, he should be able to come up with something that would work for bracing. He was employed by NASA at Langley, and I asked him if they had equipment for some metal stress tests to see why Chris was so hard on braces. Bob said that he would check into it, but he made some close observations of Chris as he walked. Bob concluded that it was not the weight on the brace that was causing it to break, it was the stress caused by metal fatigue. He went on to explain that as Chris walked with the swing-through gait, he led with his left foot and then landed in a slightly twisting motion. This action was bending or twisting the brace with each step that Chris took. It was as though one took a coat hanger in his hands and bent it back and forth, finally breaking it. Bob indicated that this had been the cause of some airplane crashes.

The next time that Chris went to see Tommy, Bob arranged to meet us in Richmond. He told Tommy what he believed the problem to be and suggested that the pelvic band be made out of spring steel so it would have some give as Chris walked. Tommy suddenly realized that Bob was probably right in this theory. He proposed another solution to the problem. Instead of the spring steel, he would simply make the band in two pieces and join it in the middle of the back with leather lacing. This technique was the way he fitted many artificial limbs. The two-piece pelvic band was most satisfactory. Tommy later began to make all braces requiring a pelvic band in this way.

The summer before Chris was to enter high school, Dr. Hammer performed surgery on Chris's clubbed feet. Several bones were almost coming through the skin on the bottom of his feet. The sores were bad, and we could not get them to heal up. For the second time he was admitted to MCV Hospital.

This time, he was placed in a beautiful room on the ninth floor with a view of the capitol and the governor's mansion. There was a studio couch for me, and the room was decorated in bright, cheerful colors. It looked more like a motel room than a hospital room. Dr. Hammer said that Chris would be hospitalized for about three weeks. The afternoon before the surgery, we settled ourselves in for a nice "vacation."

Chris tried to talk Dr. Hammer into letting him stay awake to observe the operation. Dr. Hammer replied that he didn't want to be told how to perform the operation. He knew that Chris would be talking all the time if he were awake. The operation was supposed to take several hours. I decided to go on a shopping trip while Chris was out of the room.

I wasn't gone very long, but when I returned, I found Chris sitting up in bed, reading a comic book. His feet were bound in white plastic casts propped up on pillows. Dr. Hammer had been very thoughtful when he applied the casts. He put a handle on each one, so that I could get a hold on them when I needed to lift Chris.

The second day, Dr. Hammer agreed to Chris's request that he be allowed to get up in a wheelchair. Chris was everywhere on that floor. He visited every patient, whether he was to have visitors or not. He followed the nurses as they went on their rounds. Not surprisingly, Chris was discharged the next day.

Jimmy had built a ramp at the back door of the house, so that he was able to get in and out of the house whenever he wanted. He was up and down the street all summer long. Jimmy and I often commented that he stayed outside more that summer than he had since he was a small child. Several times that summer, his Dad put him in the back of our Jeep and they went off to the lake to fish. He and his Dad had great times, but not much luck fishing. They caught only a few small ones.

Jimmy and Chris liked to fish and crab together. After the summer of the World's Fair, we decided that we could not vacation at the beach with Chris. He was not satisfied to swim in a motel pool. He wanted to get out onto the beach and into the ocean. The sand was too hot for him to crawl or slide to the water, and it would ruin a pair of braces.

We found a small resort hotel on the Rappahanock River—

an ideal vacation spot for us. There was a pool for me, a pier from which Jimmy and Chris could fish and crab, a beautiful view from the rocking-chair–lined porch, and a great abundance of exceptionally good food. We managed a week or two, there, during the summers of Chris's high school years. We made many friends during our stay at the little hotel, which was razed later to make room for more modern condominiums. We felt as though we had lost one of our friends.

By the time that Chris entered high school, I had come to the conclusion that maybe the independence we had worked so hard to build for him had been overdone. He was just like any other teenager; one day he was very dependent on his family, and the next day he didn't need anybody else's help. Physically, he was able to function completely independently. Sometimes, I was concerned that he was going to be the cause of injury to his classmates.

There were three floors in the high school building, with no elevator. Chris came down the steps four at a time, and went up at the rate of three at a time. If he should have missed a step and slid into the students that were in front of him on the steps, they would have been thrown down the steps. I guess that God was watching after the other students as well as Chris, for he never slipped when other students were around. He did admit to falling down several steps one day, when he was watching a good-looking girl going up the steps as he was going down.

Chris participated in many of the school activities. He had learned to play the trumpet when he was still in elementary school, so he joined the high school band. The band director suggested that he learn to play the French horn. He never marched with the band, but he did travel with them on some occasions. He liked to sing and became a member of the chorus when he was in eighth grade. His classes did not permit him to be full-time member after that year, but he did sing with the chorus when he had the time.

Chris worked as business manager of the school annual, after proving himself by doing a successful job of selling advertisements. The principal often said that he felt the three Grandles should go into business together. Chris should do the sales and promotion work, and Art and Bob should do the design and engineering. Chris always had had a way with people. All the kids in high school seemed to like him, and he got along well with them.

One teacher, who had just started to teach, said later that he was frightened at the thought of having Chris in his classroom. He felt that he would feel sorry for him and treat him differently from the other students. When he received his class assignments, he found that Chris had been assigned to him. He considered asking that Chris be put in another class, but being a new teacher, he was also afraid to make this request, so he began the year with Chris in his class. It did not take but a few days and some practical jokes by the kids in the class, for the teacher to find that Chris was just another one of the guys in the class. He could take the jokes and give them as well as the next kid. The fact that he had four legs instead of the normal two didn't change the fact that he was a teenage boy.

For three of his high school years he served as manager of the basketball team. He traveled with the team and managed to earn his letter in athletics in this way. As official scorekeeper, it was his responsibility to report the games to the local and nearby city papers. He was soon on a first-name basis with all of the sportswriters in the area.

In Virginia, a student can get his driver's license when he is sixteen, provided that he had been enrolled in and successfully passed a certified driver training program. Otherwise, he cannot get a permit to drive until he is eighteen. All of Chris's friends were beginning to get permits. This license is the best birthday present that most sixteen-year-olds can receive. The driver training cars at the school were not equipped with hand controls which Chris would need, nor were any of the instructors at the school certified to teach with hand controls.

During his sophomore year, Chris's classes were scheduled so that he had a free class period for about two and a half hours each Friday. He had enrolled in several science classes that had double period labs during the first part of the week. When he enrolled in these courses, he had no idea this scheduling of classes would make it possible for him to receive his driver's training. The classroom training was taught during the first part of the year as a section of the physical education classes he was required to take for graduation.

We happened to live about twenty-five miles from one of the most outstanding rehabilitation centers in the East: Woodrow Wilson Rehabilitation Center. Mom was able to arrange her schedule so that she could take Chris each Friday during his free periods to get his training.

Chris was sixteen on Sunday. . . . On Monday afternoon after we got out of school, Chris and I went to the office of the Division of Motor Vehicles for his test. He passed with flying colors and was awarded his driver's permit. During the several weeks he had been learning how to drive, we had hand controls installed on the family car. Now, he could drive it when he needed to go somewhere without me.

One evening, just before Christmas, I was returning home from a party that our church choir had at a member's home out from town. I was riding with friends. As we topped a hill headed toward town, I saw flares and lights of a state police car indicating a wreck up ahead. When we were close enough to see the accident, I suddenly spotted our little red Jeep parked nearby; then I recognized one of the mangled cars sitting in the highway as our family station wagon.

All I could think of was getting out of that car and across the road to Chris. . . . I knew he had been driving the car that evening to an annual staff meeting at school. There was Jimmy at the side of the car. Chris was not injured, just scared to death. In fact, no one was injured. There was just a lot of damage to both cars.

I learned the story piece by piece. Chris had offered to take a friend home and was driving toward the boy's home a short distance from town. He was traveling at the speed limit or slightly less, when he topped a hill and saw a car pull across the highway a short distance in front of him. Chris remembered that he was supposed to stay in his lane. He applied his brakes hard, but they just would not stop the heavy station wagon in time to avoid the crash. The other car was driven by a friend of ours who took the full blame for the accident. He said that he pulled into the highway without realizing what he was doing. Then, instead of trying to get out of the way, he applied his brakes right in front of Chris.

We were without a car for almost six weeks, but just as soon as the car was repaired, Chris was back behind the wheel. However, he became a much more cautious driver than before the accident. Maybe this was God's way of taming him a little, for a car is a necessary part of his life.

Each year, at the time for the annual prom, many of the girls in the junior and senior classes are very frustrated because they are not invited to go. The school faculty members do all that they can to persuade the guys in the class to take the girls to the dance. Some of the boys simply refuse. Bob and Art each went one year to the prom, but the second year, no amount of talking would make them decide to invite a girl to go to the prom. However, Chris invited a date to go with him to the prom both his junior and senior years. He had great fun dressed in his formal dinner jacket and black tie. When it came time to get on the dance floor, Chris and his date were right there, Chris twisting and turning to the beat of the music just like all of the other kids. There was an "after-party" and breakfast each year. Chris attended both, having as good a time as any of his classmates.

I taught in the same high school that Chris attended. I was hoping not to have him assigned to one of my classes, because I do not think that it is a good idea to have one of your own children in your class if it can possibly be avoided. Several years before, I had had Bob in my class. That worked out in a fairly satisfactory manner, because Bob has the most gentle disposition of the three boys. He is very much like his father. I don't believe Art and I could have survived a month in the same classroom, because we are so much alike, and we both tend to have quick tempers. Chris's temperament is less quick than Art's, yet he is more likely to criticize than Bob.

During his senior year, I was assigned to teach the only class of advanced math offered that year. Chris wanted to go into engineering, and he had to have that material. There was no alternative except for me to have him in my class. We managed to work it out. In some ways, it may have been a good experience, because I realized that Chris was a lazy student. During his early childhood, he had found that whenever he wanted information, he could ask his brother Bob. Bob, always very patient, sat down and explained things to Chris. Art would simply tell Chris to look it up for himself and go on his way. Then, there was also the television that Chris watched a great deal. Thus, Chris developed the habit of trying to get the information from someone instead of digging it out himself. This habit caused him problems in later years. However, he and Bob developed a very close relationship because of Bob's willingness to help him.

The time for Chris to make college applications came all too soon. It was hard to realize that eighteen years could pass so quickly. Chris was interested in attending only one school: The University of Virginia—School of Engineering and Applied Science. He applied for early decision admission and was accepted. One of the conditions of his admission was that he have a car to use at school. His high school graduation present was a little yellow Firebird. It was also his birthday present that year.

Bob and Art gave him a tape deck, which they installed for him. Later, he bought himself a scanner that Bob installed; still later, he was able to get a CB radio to add to the equipment on the car. All of the equipment needed antennas—two, long, whip antennas on the back bumper. His little Firebird looked like a mobile radio station. There was not another car in the area like it, and anyone could quickly identify Chris as he drove around town or over the campus of the University.

IX

In August 1972, we drove to Staunton to attend my aunt's funeral, and then we drove out to the interstate highway to come home. There, Chris left us in his yellow Firebird and headed in the opposite direction for Charlottesville and his years at the "university." Tears came to my eyes as I watched our youngest son go off to college. I couldn't help but reach out and take Jimmy's hand lying on the seat beside me. I knew that he felt just as I did. We both were confident that Chris would be able to live in the dormitory and get along with his roommates, but it would be rather quiet around the house in the days to come. We were both thankful that Chris had not selected a school a great distance from home. He planned to come home as many weekends as possible.

He had not been at school too long before we received a phone call: "Mom, I locked my keys in the car and I'm parked at the dining hall! What do I do?"

Naturally, I wanted to know how he could have done such a thing. He had offered a beautiful girl a ride to the dining hall. He was engaged in an interesting conversation when he got out of the car and left the keys in the switch. He locked the door as was his habit, had dinner, and then came back to find that he couldn't get back into his car. So, Jimmy got in our car and took him the extra set of keys that I kept on my key ring. Next day, we had another key made to hide on the outside of Chris's car.

A few days later, we got another call. It had been raining

for several days in Charlottesville, and there was a lot of mud around campus. "Mom, I fell in the mud and broke my crutch." Consequently, we made another trip across the mountain to take him a spare crutch that was here at the house. After a few such emergencies, Chris got most of the spare equipment to Charlottesville, and he no longer called for help, just money. I don't think he ever wrote a letter home; he just picked up the phone and called collect. He told me that it was so much easier and he could really get an answer so much more rapidly than by letter. It also took less effort; he needed the time to study. . . . So he told us.

During the summer months, he got a job working for the local recreation department as a park supervisor. His responsibilities included the supervision of some of the high school boys who worked for the department during the summer. He also checked the parking areas to see that people were not parking on the grass. He liked most the part of his job that gave him the opportunity to help people find places for picnicking or to find lost children. In fact, he was always happiest on his job when he was able to meet, talk with people, and help them in some way.

Several nights each week, he had the responsibility of locking up the city parks. I often wondered how he could lock up, for there was a heavy iron post which fit into a hole in the middle of the entrance roadway. It sat by the side of the road during the day. One night he asked me to ride with him so that he would have some company as he made the final check of the park. I was amazed at the system he had developed to get the post from the side of the roadway into the center. He stood on one crutch . . . pulled the post from its hole and put it down on the roadway in front of him. Then, he gave the post a hard push with his crutch; it slid several feet toward the center of the road. He picked the post up with one hand and positioned it in the hole. Then, he walked back and brought the gates to the center and locked them on the post. All was secure for the night.

He felt so important, one night, when the police called

him to come to the park to open the gate so that they might get in. A neighbor had reported hearing someone yelling in the area of the swimming pool. Chris was out of the house like a shot. He was out of his car and had the gates open almost before the police car arrived. Fortunately, they found nothing; no one was in trouble that night.

During the summers, he learned to know many of the younger children who were part of the playground recreation program. They loved to ride with him in his car and play with all the radios. To the young children of the community, I became known as Chris's mother.

Chris used his car, because the city recreation department vehicles were not equipped with hand controls. He furnished his own gas, but the department director paid him a little more than others with similar responsibilities, to help cover the cost of operating his car. I often joked that I thought I was paying the recreation department to let Chris work. However, the department employees often commented that Chris did a very good job of supervising the park. He took his job very seriously. He even felt that he could not take time off to come home for his meals, so the family began the practice of eating our evening meal in the park. Dinner went right into the back end of the station wagon. Each evening, Mom and I had it all spread out on the table when Jimmy came from work and Chris came around on his regular run. We learned to love the park those summers that Chris worked there. It was always so peaceful and quiet. Well, almost always.

One evening, just as we were about to finish eating, we heard a terrible crash just down the road from where we were eating; yet, the accident was around the corner, out of our view. Chris was into his car and off down the road like a streak of lightning. After some time, when he failed to return, my curiosity got the best of me, and I went to see what happened. A small car had left the roadway, traveled between two trees, and up onto a big rock. There it sat, atop the rock. The young boys who were in the car were not hurt, but the mishap caused a problem of how to get the car off of the rock. Chris called for the police and a wrecker. They finally found a solution to the situation. Chris had to supervise the entire operation to be sure that the grounds of the park did not receive further damage.

Chris's first two years of college went fairly well, although he was not the most outstanding student on campus. He was allowed to live in the dorm during his second year, and we felt that this was probably the best solution for him. He questioned us about an apartment. When his brothers were in college, they had lived in the dorms all four years. At that time, only those who took their academics lightly or had a lot of money lived in apartments. We did not realize that things had changed. We insisted that he live in the dorm his third year. He had what for most people would have seemed an ideal situation, but it was not so ideal for Chris. He was given a private room in a suite of first-year students. Chris was too interested in what his suitemates were doing; he couldn't stay in his room by himself and study as he should have. He had to be with people where the action was. That third year was almost a disaster. His grades went down; in fact, several of them hit bottom. He lost a lot of his confidence, and I was really concerned about him. By the end of that year, he made the decision to live in an apartment the next year with two guys whom he had learned to know rather well. Both were above average students. I had to laugh one day when one of Chris's professors warned that he was not to lead them astray.

This same professor got Chris interested in his thesis project. The university received a grant from the National Science Foundation for the purposes of developing electronically controlled devices for aiding the mobility of paraplegics. Chris became interested in working on electronically controlled artificial limbs. The first part of the project was assigned to Chris. He was to develop a computer program which would simulate the human body in a walking motion. This program was necessary to determine the stress and weight at the various points. This project led him to develop an interest in control devices and, as a result, a renewed interest in his studies.

The following summer, he took a class at the local college to get some of the lost credit and also to regain his confidence. The renewal effort and the apartment living seemed to be the combination that got him back on the right academic track.

During the third year, he had joined several professional organizations on campus and was elected president of one of them. The next year, he was to serve as vice-president of another. One evening, he called home to see if his Daddy could get enough turkey to serve about sixty people who were going to have an outing. His Dad told him that would be possible, but how were they going to get the turkey cooked? Well, he thought that some of the girls of the engineering school could cook it. Both Jimmy and I were a little bit afraid that the girls had never before seen that much turkey at one time, much less cooked it. So, I volunteered to cook the turkey for them. It was agreed that Chris would come home on the way to the farm to get the turkey.

He arrived a day early, with a request for the family car. It seemed they needed transportation for some of the members, and he had offered to provide it. His car would seat only two comfortably, although I have seen the time when he had five people in it.

So, he took the car back to Charlottesville, picked up the members, three girls and two boys. He said one girl was his date; then he came back home, picked up the turkey, and headed for a weekend at the river farm owned by a professor.

Late Sunday evening, he brought the car home and reported that not a bit of turkey was left. Only forty people had shown up, but they had all been very hungry.

Back to school he went in his yellow Firebird to classes the next day. At times, I have lifted the books that he carried to class. I often wondered that he could even lift them, for it took all the strength I could manage to get them up off of the floor. He carried them in a knapsack on his back, a practice of his even in elementary school.

I am amused today to see so many college students using the same method for carrying their books. When Chris first

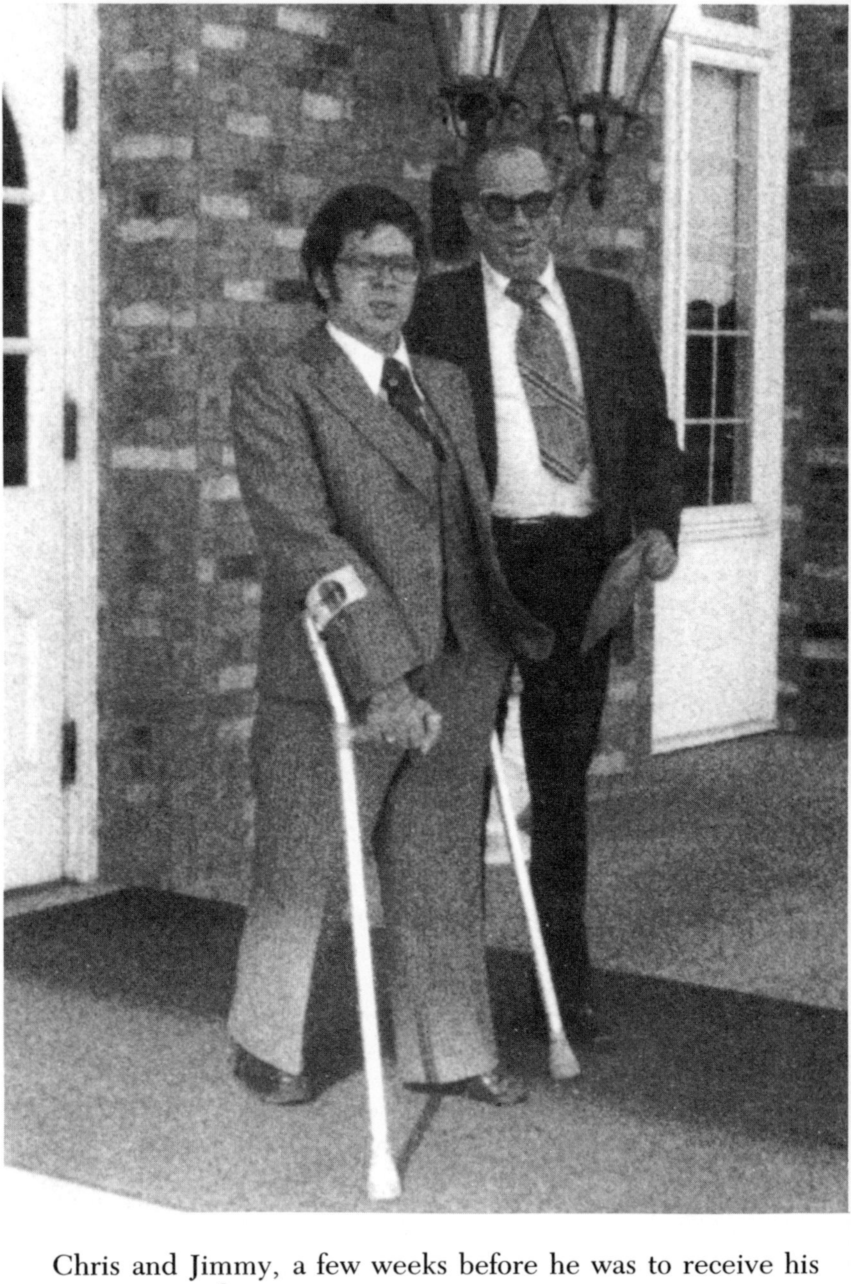

Chris and Jimmy, a few weeks before he was to receive his engineering degree.

carried books, no one ever saw a knapsack, except for carrying camping or hiking equipment. Now, knapsacks are a common scene on the American college campus. Chris was just ahead of the times, or maybe it goes back to those early remarks that I made to people when they asked if Chris would be able to do various things: "He'll be able to do anything that he wants to do; he will just have to do it in his own way!"

How quickly those years at the university passed! There we were, standing on the lawn, watching the academic procession as it moved from the Rotunda to Cabell Hall. Through my tears, I could see the rainbow with its pot of gold at the end—our Chris. I heard his name called, and watched as he walked up to receive his degree in Electrical Engineering. He was happy and a little scared as he contemplated the future, working for a large company in their components and standards division. He had decided to continue to live with us for a year or two until he was settled into his job and learned the community where he would be working. That decision made us happy, yet we know the day will soon come when he will establish a home of his own, for he is as independent as either of our other children.

God has opened many doors and led us through many dark valleys. He will continue to guide and direct our lives and that of our Chris, until His plan is fulfilled. With each tear has been a rainbow, and at its end, our pot of gold.

Epilogue

Late in July 1983, many of our friends and family gathered at a very lovely little church on top of a mountain near Alderson, West Virginia, to share in the joy that we experienced as Chris was married. His bride was radiant as she came down the aisle on her father's arm.

In the six years after his graduation from college, Chris had worked for one of the nation's largest firms as a quality control engineer. For the first year and a half he lived with us and commuted to work a distance of about twenty-five miles. It was so good to have him at home and we enjoyed his company, but it was becoming more and more obvious that he wanted to get out on his own. He wanted a place that he could say was his.

We were delighted that he asked me to help him in his search for a home near his work. Jimmy and I felt that a condominium would be the most suitable because of the maintenance, et cetera. Chris did not agree. "That would be too much like living in an apartment." He wanted a house.

Finally, he found a house that he liked, even though Jimmy and I wondered about how he would get along. There were long, steep steps leading to the basement laundry room. That would been no problem, he assured us, if Jimmy would just put up a rail along the side of the steps. The laundry went up and down on his back in his knapsack.

I was surprised at his housekeeping ability. He tried cooking, but decided that cooking for one was not much fun and that he could eat out just about as cheaply as he could cook for himself.

After about two years in that first home, he was transferred to another city in Virginia, where he found another house. Several times, he made the remark to me that he felt that he would like to have a wife to share his life. He had many friends, but he felt that was just not what he wanted.

Chris joined a singles group, went to church, and joined other groups where he thought that he might meet "that right person." All to no avail.

One day, he mentioned the fact to his boss that he just had not met any young women that he enjoyed being with more than a time or two. His boss suggested that he try a dating service. Together, they went through the "Yellow Pages" of the local phone book and found a dating service listed.

Chris applied to the service and he was supposed to get the names of five dates for 35 dollars. On the application, he indicated that he would be willing to travel a maximum of a hundred miles.

As fate would have it, the first name that he received was that of a young lady that lived just about a hundred miles away in a little town in West Virginia. Chris and Becky met for their first date by the telephone booth in front of the County Court House where they would, in time, get their marriage license.

We didn't see much of Chris during the fall and winter of 1982, so we weren't really surprised when they came to see us one weekend to show off the shiny new diamond ring on Becky's third finger—left hand.

On Palm Sunday, Becky's parents, Jimmy and I, and Mother took dinner, and all met for the first time at Chris's home. It seemed that we had know each other for years, instead of just meeting for the first time. The two fathers discovered that they had many things in common, as did Becky's mother and I. So, from there the plans went forth for their wedding day, July 30, 1983.

After a short honeymoon at the Greenbrier Hotel, they went home to the house that Chris had been living in alone.

When Chris first moved into his own home, I felt that I needed to call him each morning to be sure that he was all right. I think that I really bugged him when I did this, because he finally told me that he was getting up early and meeting some of the fellows from work for breakfast. . . . I still worried.

I no longer feel the need to call Becky and Chris each morning, although we do talk to each other frequently. I now have a daughter to love and look after Chris.

God has truly filled our POT OF GOLD to the brim.